THE LOW-FODMAP DIET FOR BEGINNERS

A 28-Day Plan to Beat Bloat and Soothe Your Gut with Tasty Recipes and Bonus Symptom Tracker Included

Stephen William

Table Of Contents

Section 1: Introduction to FODMAPs	01-04
Section 2: Preparing for Your FODMAP Journey	05-11
Section 3: The 28-Day FODMAP Meal Plan	11-12
Week 1	15-34
WeeK 1 reflection	35-36
Week 2	37-58
WeeK 2 reflection	59-60
Week 3	61-82
WeeK 3 reflection	83-84
Week 4	85-106
WeeK 4 Reflection	107-108
FODMAP Journey Progress Table	109-137
Section 4: What Next	139-144

LOW FODMAP DIET, 28 DAYS TO HEAL THE GUT

Welcome aboard the FODMAP Express, a 28-day gastronomic journey designed to transform your relationship with food and your gut. This book isn't just a collection of recipes; it's your passport to a world where food is both delicious and gut-friendly, taking you from bloated and bewildered to blissful and balanced.

What's Cooking Inside:

- The FODMAP Voyage: Set sail on the sea of FODMAP knowledge, navigating through what it is, why it matters, and how it can be your lighthouse to gut health.
- Symptom Spotting & Solutions: Learn to be the detective in your digestive story, identifying the sneaky culprits behind discomfort and how to outsmart them with food.
- 28-Day Delicious Detour: Each day is a new culinary adventure, with meals designed not just to satisfy your taste buds but also to bring peace to your digestive realm.
- Reflection week by week of your progress so far
- What to do next

SECTION 1: INTRODUCTION TO FODMAPS

The low FODMAP diet is a temporary eating plan that's very restrictive

The FODMAP Landscape: Understanding What FODMAPs Are

Welcome to the fascinating world of FODMAPs - a landscape populated by a diverse array of foods that can either be comforting or challenging for your digestive system. The term FODMAP stands for Fermentable Oligosaccharides, Disaccharides, Monosaccharides, and Polyols. These are short-chain carbohydrates and sugar alcohols found in various foods, and for some, they're like uninvited guests causing turmoil in their digestive tract.

Imagine your gut as a bustling city where different foods come to visit. Most are like friendly tourists, contributing positively to the city's vibe. But FODMAPs can be likened to tourists who unintentionally stir trouble, leading to uncomfortable digestive symptoms for those sensitive to them.

The FODMAP journey is unique for each person. For some, consuming these carbohydrates is a non-issue; their bodies can welcome and process these visitors without any problems. However, for others with a sensitive digestive system, these carbohydrates are poorly absorbed in the small intestine. When they travel to the large intestine, they become fodder for the resident bacteria, which ferment them. This fermentation process can cause a range of symptoms, including bloating, gas, abdominal pain, and alterations in bowel habits.

Understanding FODMAPs is crucial because it offers a new perspective on managing digestive health. It's about knowing which foods to invite into your gut-city and which to limit. The key is not to eliminate FODMAPs entirely but to identify the specific types and amounts that your body can handle.
The variety of foods that fall under the FODMAP umbrella is broad. They include certain fruits, such as apples and pears; vegetables like onions and garlic; dairy products rich in lactose; wheat and other grains; and legumes. The complexity of this group makes it essential to approach the FODMAP diet methodically, as it's not about blanket elimination but rather a nuanced understanding of what works for your body.

Why FODMAP Matters: The Link Between FODMAPs and Digestive Health

Have you ever finished a meal only to feel like your stomach has turned into a balloon ready to take flight? This discomfort can often be attributed to FODMAPs, especially in individuals with a sensitive digestive system. The relationship between FODMAPs and digestive health is a critical piece of the puzzle for those experiencing gastrointestinal distress.

For those with sensitivities, undigested FODMAPs make their way to the large intestine, where they become a feast for gut bacteria. This bacterial banquet results in excessive fermentation, producing gas and attracting water into the gut. This process can lead to symptoms like bloating, abdominal pain, gas, diarrhea, and constipation. It's akin to having a rowdy party in your gut, where the guests overstay their welcome, causing chaos and discomfort.

The significance of FODMAPs in managing digestive health cannot be overstated. By identifying and modifying your intake of these fermentable carbohydrates, you can transform your digestive experiences. The goal is not to wage a war against these foods but to understand your body's unique responses to them. This understanding can help you sculpt a diet that keeps your gut flora balanced and your digestive system running smoothly.

For individuals with conditions like Irritable Bowel Syndrome (IBS) or Small Intestinal Bacterial Overgrowth (SIBO), the low FODMAP diet is particularly relevant. Studies have shown that up to 86% of people with IBS experience relief from their symptoms when following this diet. The diet's effectiveness lies in its ability to help identify which foods are problematic for the individual and to create a personalized eating plan that minimizes gastrointestinal distress.

Embarking on a low FODMAP diet is a journey of discovery. It involves understanding the intricate relationship between what you eat and how you feel. This journey isn't about deprivation; it's about empowerment and learning to make food choices that support your digestive health. With each step, you move closer to a life where your meals bring you nourishment and joy, rather than discomfort and anxiety.

Decoding the Digestive Dilemma: Symptoms and Conditions Associated with FODMAP Sensitivities

When your gut sends out an SOS, it's crucial to listen. This distress signal can manifest in various forms - bloating, gas, stomach cramps, diarrhea, constipation, and more. These symptoms are the body's way of signaling that something isn't quite right in the digestive system. Understanding and responding to these signals is the essence of managing FODMAP sensitivities.

Irritable Bowel Syndrome (IBS) and Small Intestinal Bacterial Overgrowth (SIBO) are two conditions often linked with FODMAP sensitivities. IBS, a common disorder affecting the large intestine, can cause a constellation of symptoms including cramping, abdominal pain, bloating, gas, and changes in bowel habits. SIBO, on the other hand, occurs when there is an abnormal increase in the overall bacterial population in the small intestine, especially types of bacteria not typically found in that part of the digestive tract.

For those with IBS or SIBO, FODMAPs can be the hidden triggers of their symptoms. When these fermentable carbohydrates are poorly absorbed in the small intestine, they make their way to the large intestine where they are fermented by bacteria, producing gas and drawing water into the intestine. This can exacerbate the symptoms of IBS and SIBO, leading to significant discomfort.

The process of decoding this digestive dilemma begins with identifying the relationship between your symptoms and your intake of FODMAPs. This is where the low FODMAP diet comes into play. By systematically eliminating high FODMAP foods and then gradually reintroducing them, you can identify which specific foods trigger your symptoms. This personalized approach allows you to tailor your diet to your body's needs, avoiding foods that trigger symptoms while enjoying those that don't.

In this section, we will dive into the various symptoms associated with FODMAP sensitivities and the conditions they are linked with. We'll explore how to effectively use the low FODMAP diet as a tool for symptom management and how to integrate this knowledge into a sustainable, enjoyable eating plan. By understanding the foods that work best with your body, you can embark on a path to improved gut health and overall wellbeing.

SECTION 2: PREPARING FOR YOUR FODMAP JOURNEY

Setting the Stage: Mental and Physical Preparation for the 28-Day Plan

Embarking on a 28-day journey with the FODMAP plan is akin to preparing for a transformative expedition into your dietary habits and health. This journey demands not just an understanding of what you'll eat, but also a readiness of your environment and mindset.

By failing to prepare, you are preparing to fail

1. ASSESSING YOUR ENVIRONMENT: CREATING A FODMAP-FRIENDLY SPACE

The first step in your FODMAP journey is to ensure your environment supports your dietary changes. This involves making your kitchen a place that aligns with your new eating plan:

- **Audit Your Pantry and Fridge:** Go through your current food supplies and identify high-FODMAP foods. Familiarize yourself with common high-FODMAP ingredients like wheat, dairy products high in lactose, certain fruits like apples and pears, and vegetables like onions and garlic.
- **Remove Temptations:** Clear out items that are high in FODMAPs. This helps prevent accidental consumption of foods that could trigger symptoms.
- **Restock with Alternatives:** Replace the removed items with low-FODMAP alternatives. For example, choose lactose-free dairy products, gluten-free grains, and FODMAP-friendly fruits and vegetables like oranges, grapes, carrots, and potatoes.
- **Organize for Accessibility:** Arrange your kitchen so that low-FODMAP foods are easily accessible. This can make meal preparation quicker and less stressful.
- **Create a FODMAP Information Center:** Consider having a section in your kitchen where you can keep FODMAP guides, lists of suitable foods, and recipes. This can serve as a quick reference point while cooking or planning meals.

2. CRAFTING A MINDFUL EATING SPACE

Creating a mindful eating environment is crucial in helping you tune into your body's cues and enjoy your meals without distraction.

- Choose a Dedicated Eating Area: Select a specific spot in your home for eating. This should be away from high-traffic areas and distractions like the TV or computer. A quiet corner in your dining room or a space with a view of the outdoors can be ideal.
- Minimize Distractions: Ensure this space is free from electronic distractions. Eating without the interference of screens allows you to focus on the act of eating and listen to your body's signals.
- Create a Comfortable Setting: Make your dining area as comfortable as possible. Comfortable seating, pleasant lighting, and a clean, organized table setting can enhance the eating experience.
- Practice Mindful Eating Techniques: Before you begin eating, take a few deep breaths to center yourself. As you eat, pay attention to the flavors, textures, and aromas of your food. Chew slowly and pause between bites. This not only aids digestion but also helps you recognize when you are full, preventing overeating.
- Listen to Your Body: Be attentive to how different foods make you feel during and after eating. This awareness is key in identifying foods that work well for you and those that don't.

2. CRAFTING A MINDFUL EATING SPACE

Setting clear, specific, and achievable goals is a vital step in your FODMAP journey, and the practice of writing them down and reviewing them daily is rooted in several psychological and practical principles:

Writing down your goals acts as a physical manifestation of your commitment. When you see your objectives in writing, it makes them more real and tangible. This process psychologically reinforces your commitment to these goals and holds you accountable. It's a daily reminder of what you're working towards and why you started this journey in the first place.

Daily review of your written goals helps keep them at the forefront of your mind. This constant reinforcement helps maintain focus on your objectives amidst the distractions of daily life. When your goals are clear and continuously in your thoughts, you're more likely to make decisions that align with achieving them.

Regularly looking at your goals enables you to visualize achieving them. Visualization is a powerful tool that can motivate and inspire you to take the necessary actions to reach your objectives. When you can clearly envision the outcome – such as feeling less bloated or having more energy – it fuels your motivation to pursue these goals.

Written goals are like milestones on a map. They allow you to measure your progress and see how far you've come since you started. This can be incredibly encouraging, especially on days when the journey feels challenging. Seeing progress, even in small steps, can boost your morale and motivate you to continue.

With your goals in writing, it becomes easier to reflect on them and assess their relevance and realism as you progress on your FODMAP journey. This reflection can lead to necessary adjustments, ensuring that your goals remain relevant and achievable as your journey evolves.

4. MENTAL READINESS: EMBRACING CHANGE AND CHALLENGES

Cultivate a Growth Mindset

- **Embrace Challenges:** View potential challenges not as obstacles, but as opportunities to learn and grow. Remind yourself that each challenge is a chance to better understand your body and what works for you.
- **Reframe Negative Thoughts:** When you encounter a setback or a difficult day, try to reframe negative thoughts into positive ones. For example, if you're feeling frustrated by a certain dietary restriction, remind yourself of the long-term benefits this change could bring to your health.

Practice Positive Self-Talk:

- **Daily Affirmations:** Start each day with positive affirmations related to your journey. For example, "I am capable of making healthy choices," or "Each step I take brings me closer to better health."
- **Replace 'Can't' with 'Can':** Whenever you find yourself thinking, "I can't have this food," switch it to, "I can find a delicious alternative that supports my health."

Set Up a Support System:

- **Seek Support:** Talk to friends, family, or online communities about your journey. Sharing your experiences and hearing others' stories can be incredibly motivating.
- **Professional Guidance:** If possible, consider sessions with a dietitian or a counselor who specializes in dietary changes. They can offer expert advice and emotional support.

Regularly Revisit Your 'Why':

As talked about previously, keep the written note or a visual representation of why you're undertaking this journey in a place you see regularly.

5. REFLECTIONS: CHARTING YOUR PROGRESS AT THE END OF EACH WEEK

At the conclusion of each week on your FODMAP journey, it's essential to pause and take stock of the changes and discoveries you've made. These weekly reflections act as your personal checkpoints, helping you to map out how your body is responding to the dietary changes. Think of it as taking a moment to gaze at the landscape you've traversed, noting the changes in terrain and how you've adapted to them.

Each week, you'll engage in a reflective practice, using a simple yet insightful rating system. This system allows you to evaluate various aspects of your health and well-being on a scale from 1 to 10, where 1 indicates 'no improvement' and 10 signifies 'significant improvement'. The aspects you'll reflect on include Digestive Comfort, Energy Levels, Sleep Quality, Mood and Mental Clarity, Physical Comfort and Pain Levels, Skin Health, Cravings and Appetite Control, and Overall Well-being.

This practice is akin to drawing a map of your journey, with each week adding more detail and depth. It's an opportunity to connect with your body's responses to the diet, offering insights into what works and what doesn't. Have you noticed a shift in your energy levels? Are you sleeping better? Is there a change in how you feel physically and mentally? These reflections are critical in understanding the unique language of your body and how it interacts with food.

By charting your progress weekly, you're not just observing changes; you're actively participating in your journey towards better health. This reflective process is a powerful tool in your journey, enabling you to tailor the FODMAP plan to your body's needs. It ensures that your path is not just guided by a set plan but is dynamically shaped by your personal experiences and insights.

As you move from one week to the next, these reflections will build a comprehensive picture of your journey. They'll help you to make informed decisions, fine-tune your diet, and understand the long-term impact of the changes you're making. Embrace these weekly reflections as a vital part of your FODMAP adventure, charting a course towards a healthier, happier you.

LABEL LITERACY: LEARNING TO READ AND UNDERSTAND FOOD LABELS

Navigating the world of food labels is a critical skill for anyone on the FODMAP journey. Understanding these labels helps you make informed choices about the foods you consume, ensuring they align with your dietary needs. Here's a breakdown of how to effectively read and understand food labels:

For managing your FODMAP intake effectively, there are several free apps you can consider:

- **Spoonful App**: This app helps determine if foods with small amounts of high FODMAP ingredients are safe to eat. It's particularly useful for understanding portion sizes, which is crucial since even high FODMAP foods may be safe in small quantities.

- **FODMAP A to Z**: This app is a handy reference for quickly checking which foods are low or high in FODMAPs. Created by an IBS patient, it features a database of around 650 everyday ingredients, helping you identify safe foods.
- **Fast FODMAP Lookup & Learn**: This app focuses on speed and accuracy for identifying FODMAP content in ingredients. It uses learning games to help remember which ingredients are high or low in FODMAPs, although it doesn't offer a complete program.

1. Start with the Ingredients List:
- **Look for FODMAPs**: Scan the ingredients for high-FODMAP items. Common culprits include garlic, onion, wheat, honey, high-fructose corn syrup, and certain dairy products.
- **Order of Ingredients**: Ingredients are listed in order of quantity, from highest to lowest. If a high-FODMAP ingredient is near the top of the list, it's best to avoid that product.
- **Hidden FODMAPs**: Be aware of less obvious FODMAP sources, like inulin, agave nectar, or chicory root, which are often found in processed foods.

2. Understanding Food Additives:
- **Identify Additives**: Some additives can be high in FODMAPs. Look out for additives like polyols (sorbitol, mannitol, xylitol), often found in sugar-free products.
- **Natural vs. Artificial Flavors**: Natural flavors can sometimes be derived from high-FODMAP sources. If you're particularly sensitive, it might be safer to choose products without these ambiguous ingredients.

3. Decoding Nutritional Information:
- **Serving Size and Servings Per Container**: Pay attention to the serving size and how many servings are in the package. This affects the FODMAP content and how much of the product is safe to consume.
- **Check for Sugars and Fiber**: Look at the sugar and fiber content. Foods high in fructose or with a high ratio of fructose to glucose can be problematic. Also, be wary of foods with high amounts of added fibers, which can be high in FODMAPs.

4. Recognizing Low FODMAP Certification Labels:
- **Certification Symbols**: Some products may carry a low FODMAP certification symbol. These products have been tested and are certified to be low in FODMAPs, which can save you time and guesswork.

5. Understanding Health Claims:
- **Misleading Claims**: Be cautious of health claims like "natural," "organic," or "gluten-free." While these might indicate a healthier product, they don't necessarily mean low FODMAP.
- **Gluten-Free Products**: For those with wheat sensitivity, gluten-free products can be a good option, but they still might contain other high-FODMAP ingredients.

6. Allergen Information:
- **Check for Allergens**: Allergen labeling can be helpful. For example, if a product says it contains dairy or wheat, it can be a signal to check more closely for high FODMAP ingredients.

7. Practice and Patience:
- **Regular Practice**: The more you read labels, the more familiar you'll become with common high and low FODMAP ingredients.
- **Keep Updated**: FODMAP research is ongoing, and food products change. Regularly updating your knowledge is key.

SECTION 3: THE 28-DAY FODMAP MEAL PLAN

Holistic Focus: Nourishing Your Overall Health
The FODMAP meal plan focuses not just on symptom alleviation but also on overall nutritional balance and wellness. It's designed to support your entire health, considering both physical and mental well-being.

The Structure: A Detailed Daily Guide
- Daily Meals: Each day includes planned meals - breakfast, lunch, dinner, along with options for snacks and drinks. All are tailored to be low in FODMAPs, catering to your dietary needs.
- Variety and Balance: The plan ensures a diverse range of foods to keep your diet interesting and nutritionally complete.
- Practicality: Meals are designed to be easy to prepare with accessible ingredients, making it convenient to
- stick to the diet.

The Goals: Aiming for Positive Outcomes
- **Symptom Relief:** The primary aim is to reduce common IBS symptoms like bloating, abdominal discomfort, and irregular bowel movements.
- **Gut Health Improvement:** The diet aims to promote a balanced gut environment, discouraging conditions that trigger IBS symptoms.
- **Lifestyle Integration:** The plan is designed to help you seamlessly incorporate these dietary changes into your daily life for long-term management.

Expected Outcomes
- **Symptom Reduction:** Anticipate a decrease in the frequency and intensity of IBS symptoms as you progress through the plan.
- **Increased Understanding:** Gain insights into how different foods affect your symptoms and overall well-being.
- **Long-Term Strategies:** By the end of the 28 days, you should have a clearer understanding of managing your symptoms through diet.

The Importance of Consistency and Adaptation
- **Following the Plan:** Consistency is key. It's essential to stick to the low FODMAP guidelines to see the full benefits.
- **Listening to Your Body:** Individual responses can vary, so it's important to note how your body reacts to different foods and adjust accordingly.
- **Patience in the Process:** Remember, changing dietary habits and seeing improvements in gut health is a gradual process. Patience and perseverance are crucial.

By adhering to this tailored 28-day low FODMAP meal plan, you're not only managing symptoms but also taking a significant step towards long-term digestive health and overall well-being. This journey is about learning what works best for your body within the framework of a low FODMAP diet and adapting these learnings into your lifestyle for sustainable health benefits.

WEEK 1: THE FODMAP LANDSCAPE - BEGINNING YOUR JOURNEY

"Welcome to Week 1 of your FODMAP journey - 'The FODMAP Landscape'. This week is all about embarking on a new path, understanding the basics of FODMAPs, and gently introducing your body to this transformative dietary approach. As you navigate through these initial days, remember that every step is a move towards a healthier gut and a happier you. Let's explore this new landscape together, discovering how these changes can begin to improve your digestive health."

> DAY 1

GREEK YOGURT PARFAIT WITH STRAWBERRIES AND ALMONDS

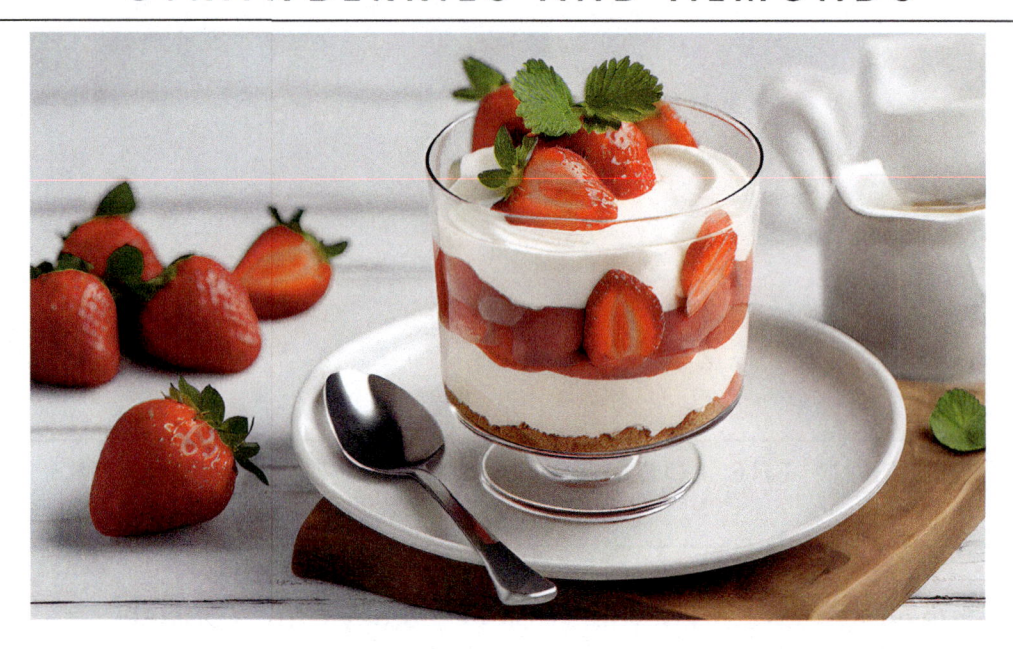

Vibe : A delightful and nutritious parfait that's gentle on the stomach.

Ingredients

1 cup lactose-free Greek yogurt
1/2 cup strawberries, sliced
2 tablespoons slivered almonds

Steps for Cooking:

1. In a glass or bowl, layer half of the Greek yogurt.
2. Add half of the sliced strawberries on top of the yogurt.
3. Sprinkle a tablespoon of slivered almonds over the strawberries.
4. Repeat the layers with the remaining ingredients.
5. Finish with a few strawberry slices and a sprinkle of almonds on top.
6. Enjoy this Low FODMAP Greek yogurt parfait for a creamy and fruity treat.

GRILLED CHICKEN SALAD WITH MIXED GREENS, CUCUMBER, AND A LEMON VINAIGRETTE

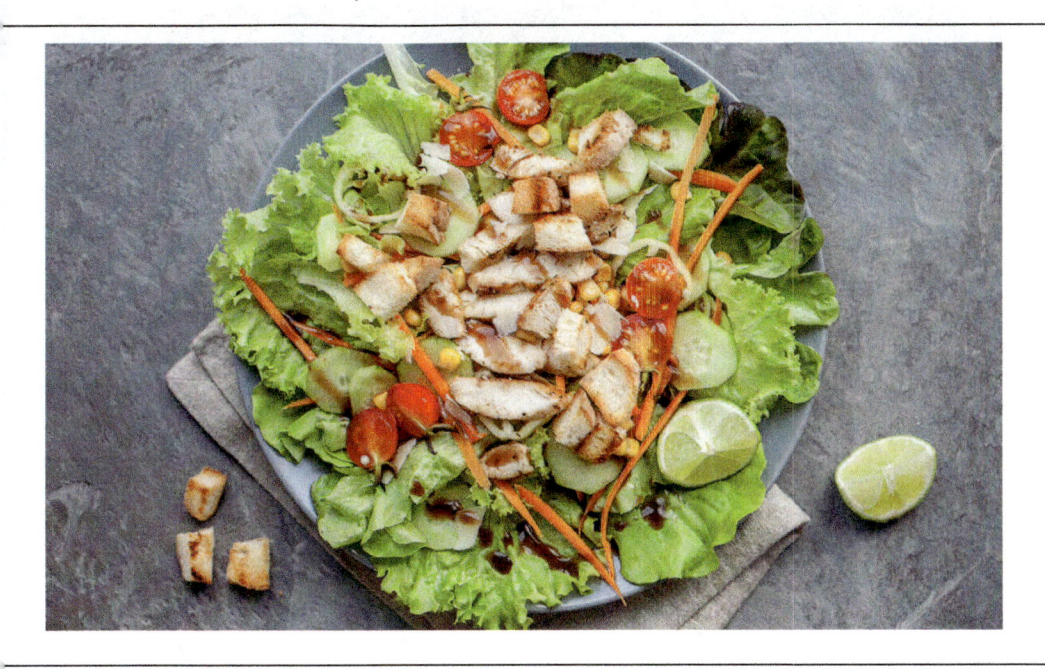

Vibe: A refreshing and protein-packed grilled chicken salad with zesty lemon vinaigrette.

Ingredients

- 4 oz grilled chicken breast, sliced
- Mixed greens (e.g., spinach, arugula, lettuce)
- 1/2 cucumber, sliced
- Lemon vinaigrette (lemon juice, olive oil, salt, and pepper)
- parmesan cheese
- add small serving off lemon vinegar

Steps for Cooking:

1. Arrange the mixed greens on a plate.
2. Top with sliced grilled chicken and cucumber.
3. Drizzle with lemon vinaigrette.
4. Toss to combine and enjoy your Low FODMAP grilled chicken salad.

BAKED SALMON WITH ROASTED CARROTS AND QUINOA

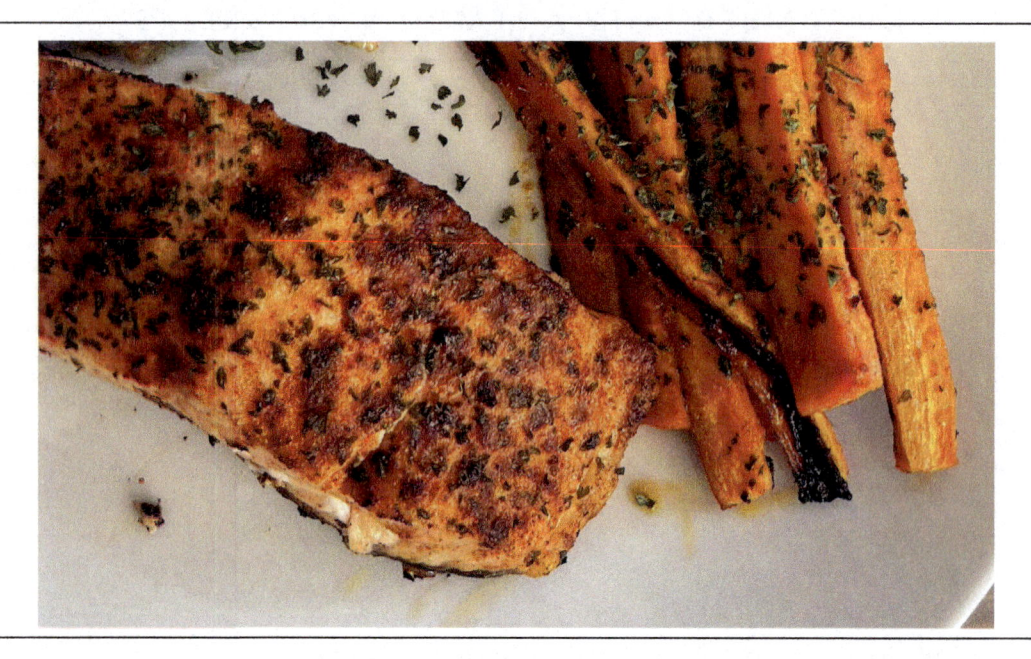

Vibe: A wholesome dinner featuring baked salmon, roasted carrots, and quinoa.

Ingredients

- Salmon fillet
- Carrot sticks, roasted
- Quinoa (check for FODMAP content)
- Olive oil, salt, and pepper for seasoning
- Lemon wedges
- Rosemary

Steps for Cooking:

1. Preheat the oven to 375°F (190°C).
2. Season salmon fillet with olive oil, Rosemary, salt, and pepper.
3. Bake salmon for about 15-20 minutes or until it flakes easily with a fork.
4. Roast carrot sticks until caramelized and tender.
5. Prepare quinoa according to package instructions (use a Low FODMAP variety).
6. Serve baked salmon with roasted carrots and quinoa.
7. Garnish with lemon wedges.
8. Enjoy your Low FODMAP baked salmon with roasted carrots and quinoa.

DAY 2

SCRAMBLED EGGS WITH SPINACH AND CHERRY TOMATOES

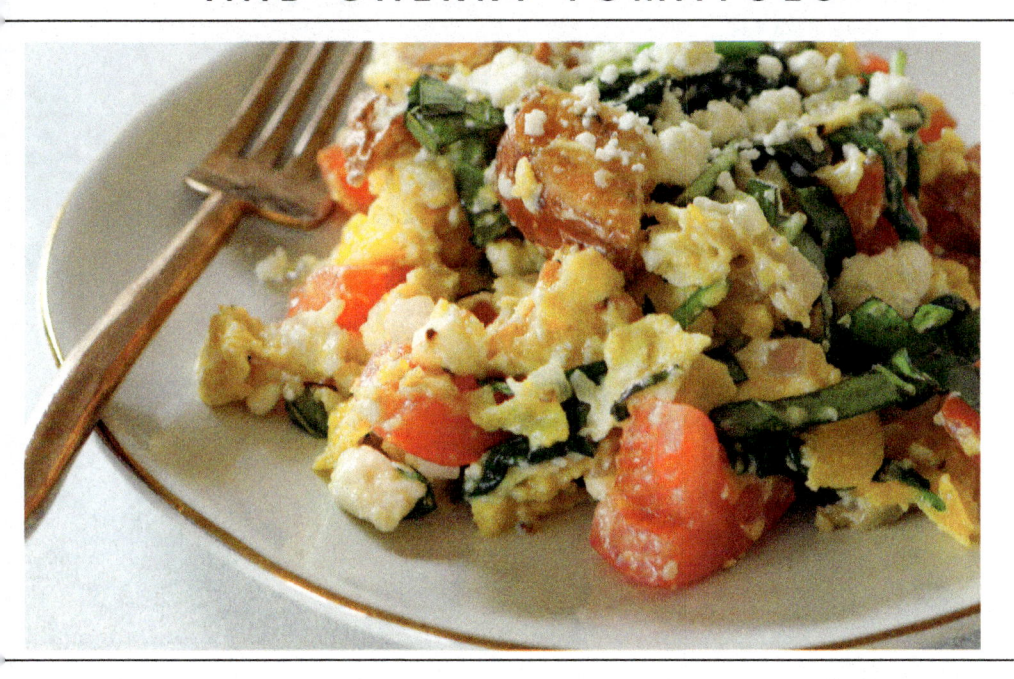

Vibe: A hearty and satisfying breakfast to kickstart your day while staying Low FODMAP.

Ingredients

- 2 large eggs
- 1 cup fresh spinach leaves
- 1/2 cup cherry tomatoes, halved
- Salt and pepper to taste
- Olive oil for cooking

Steps for Cooking:

1. Heat a non-stick skillet over medium heat and add a drizzle of olive oil.
2. In a bowl, whisk the eggs until well beaten.
3. Add spinach leaves to the skillet and sauté for a minute until they wilt.
4. Pour the beaten eggs into the skillet with the wilted spinach.
5. Stir gently as the eggs start to set.
6. Once the eggs are almost cooked through, add cherry tomato halves.
7. Continue to cook until the eggs are fully set and the tomatoes are warmed through.
8. Season with salt and pepper to taste.
9. Serve hot and enjoy your Low FODMAP scrambled eggs.

TURKEY AND CHEESE LETTUCE WRAPS WITH A SIDE OF CARROT STICKS

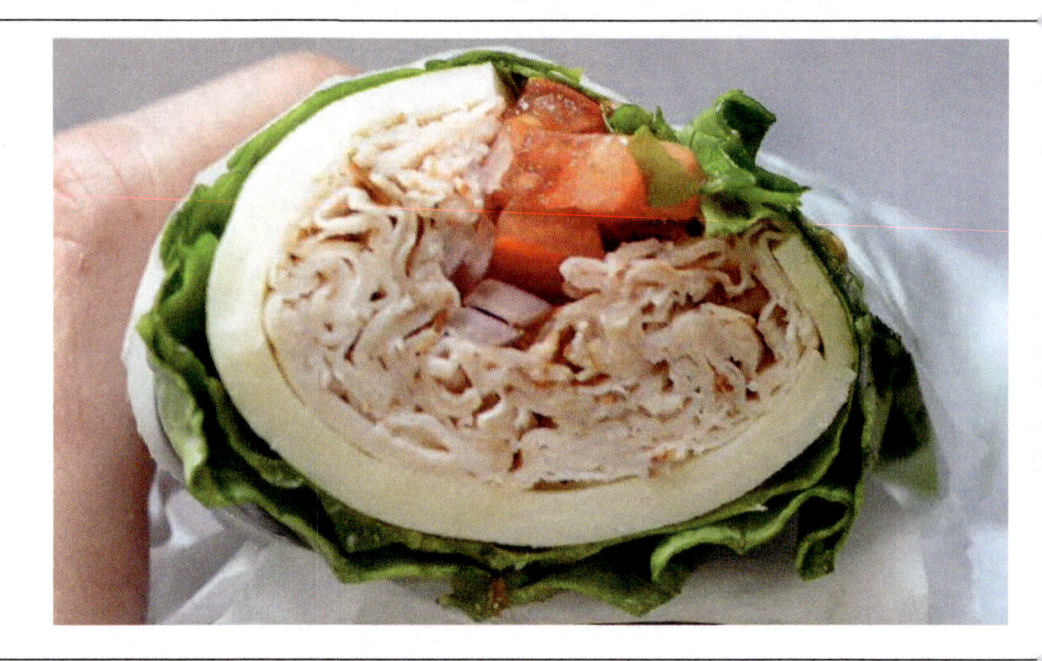

Vibe: A light and satisfying lunch with turkey and creamy avocado wrapped in lettuce leaves.

Ingredients

- large lettuce leaves (e.g., iceberg or butter lettuce)
- Cooked turkey slices
- Cheese and tomatoes
- Carrot sticks for a side

Steps for Cooking:

1. Lay out the lettuce leaves.
2. Place cooked turkey slices on each lettuce leaf.
3. Top with sliced cheese and tomatoes
4. Roll up the lettuce leaves to create wraps.
5. Serve with carrot sticks on the side.
6. Enjoy your Low FODMAP turkey and lettuce wraps.

GRILLED PORK TENDERLOIN WITH MASHED POTATOES (USING LACTOSE-FREE MILK) AND GREEN BEANS

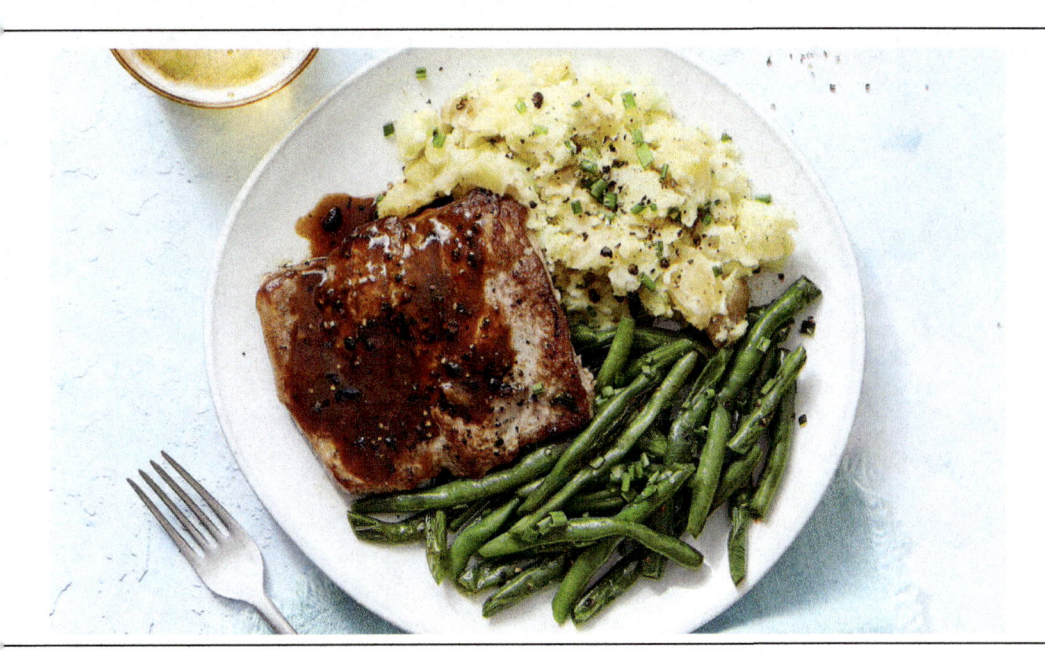

Vibe: A hearty dinner with grilled pork tenderloin, creamy mashed potatoes made with lactose-free milk, and green beans.

Ingredients

- Grilled pork tenderloin
- Potatoes (check for FODMAP content)
- Lactose-free milk
- Olive oil, salt, and pepper for seasoning
- Green beans

Steps for Cooking:

1. Grill pork tenderloin until cooked to your liking.
2. Peel and boil potatoes until tender.
3. Mash potatoes with lactose-free milk, olive oil, salt, and pepper until creamy.
4. Steam green beans until tender.
5. Serve grilled pork tenderloin with creamy mashed potatoes and green beans.
6. Enjoy your Low FODMAP grilled pork tenderloin with mashed potatoes and green beans.

DAY 3

OMELET WITH BELL PEPPERS, CHEDDAR CHEESE, AND CHIVES (GREEN PART)

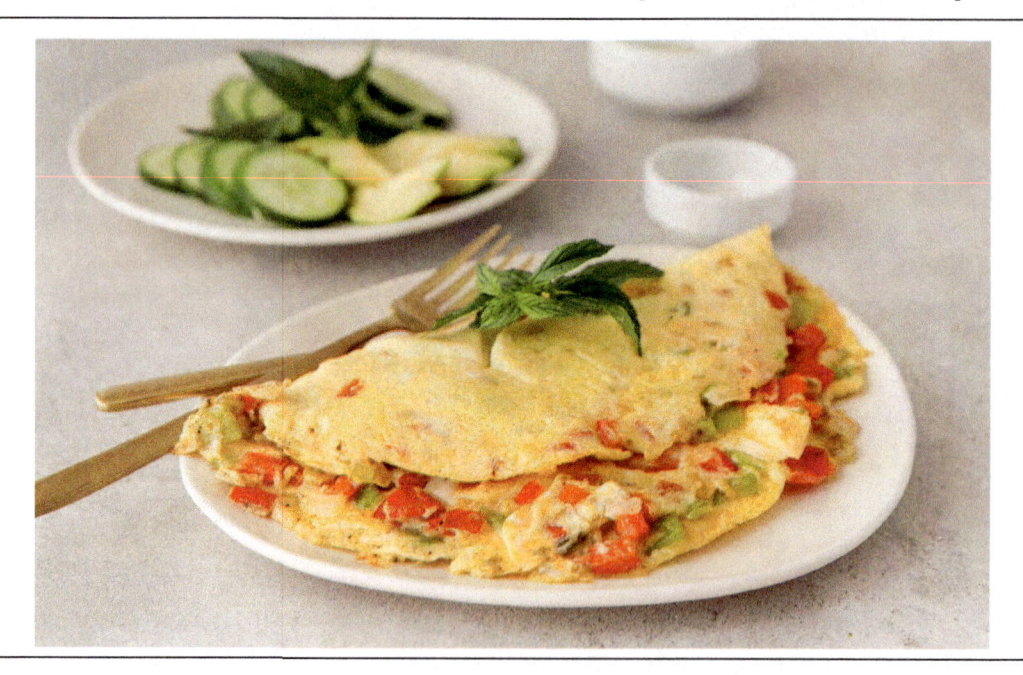

Vibe: A savory and satisfying omelet that's gentle on the tummy.

Ingredients

- 2 large eggs
- 1/4 cup red or green bell peppers, diced
- 1/4 cup cheddar cheese, grated
- Chives (green part), finely chopped, for garnish
- Salt and pepper to taste
- Olive oil for cooking

Steps for Cooking:

1. In a bowl, whisk the eggs until well beaten.
2. Heat a non-stick skillet over medium heat and add a drizzle of olive oil.
3. Add diced bell peppers to the skillet and sauté until slightly softened.
4. Pour the beaten eggs into the skillet with the sautéed peppers.
5. Sprinkle grated cheddar cheese evenly over the eggs.
6. Cook until the eggs are set and the cheese is melted.
7. Season with salt and pepper to taste.
8. Garnish with chopped chives.
9. Fold the omelet in half and transfer to a plate.
10. Serve hot and savor your Low FODMAP omelette

QUINOA SALAD WITH ROASTED RED PEPPERS, OLIVES, AND FETA CHEESE

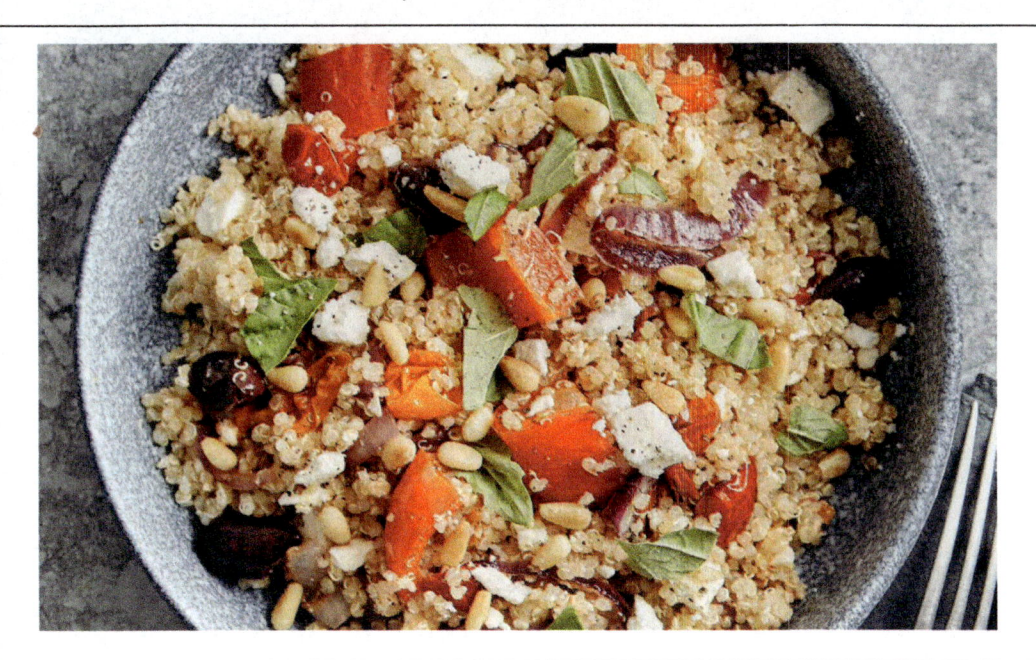

Vibe: A Mediterranean-inspired quinoa salad with bold flavors and wholesome ingredients.

Ingredients

- 1 cup cooked quinoa (check for FODMAP content)
- Roasted red peppers, diced
- Olives, sliced, cherry tomatoes
- Feta cheese (check for FODMAP content)
- Olive oil and balsamic vinegar (for dressing)
- Salt and pepper to taste

Steps for Cooking:

1. In a bowl, combine cooked quinoa, diced roasted red peppers, sliced green olives, and crumbled feta cheese.
2. Drizzle with olive oil and balsamic vinegar.
3. Season with salt and pepper to taste.
4. Toss to combine and enjoy your Low FODMAP quinoa salad.

SPAGHETTI SQUASH WITH GROUND TURKEY AND A TOMATO-BASED SAUCE (WITHOUT ONIONS AND GARLIC)

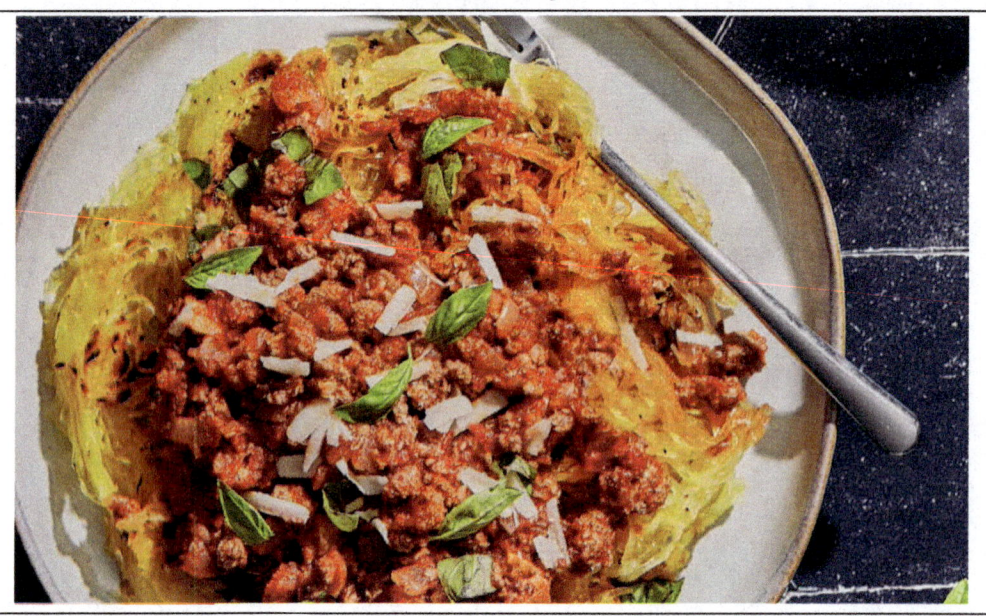

Vibe: A satisfying spaghetti squash dish with ground turkey and a tomato-based sauce.

Ingredients

- Spaghetti squash
- Ground turkey
- Tomato-based sauce (check for FODMAP content, use one without onions and garlic)
- Olive oil, salt, and pepper for seasoning

Steps for Cooking:

1. Preheat the oven to 375°F (190°C).
2. Cut the spaghetti squash in half lengthwise and remove the seeds.
3. Place squash halves cut side down on a baking sheet and roast for about 40-45 minutes or until the flesh can be easily scraped into "spaghetti" strands with a fork.
4. In a skillet, cook ground turkey in olive oil until browned.
5. Add tomato-based sauce (use one without onions and garlic) and simmer until heated through.
6. Season with salt and pepper.
7. Serve the tomato sauce over the roasted spaghetti squash.

DAY 4

QUINOA PORRIDGE WITH SLICED KIWI AND A DRIZZLE OF MAPLE SYRUP

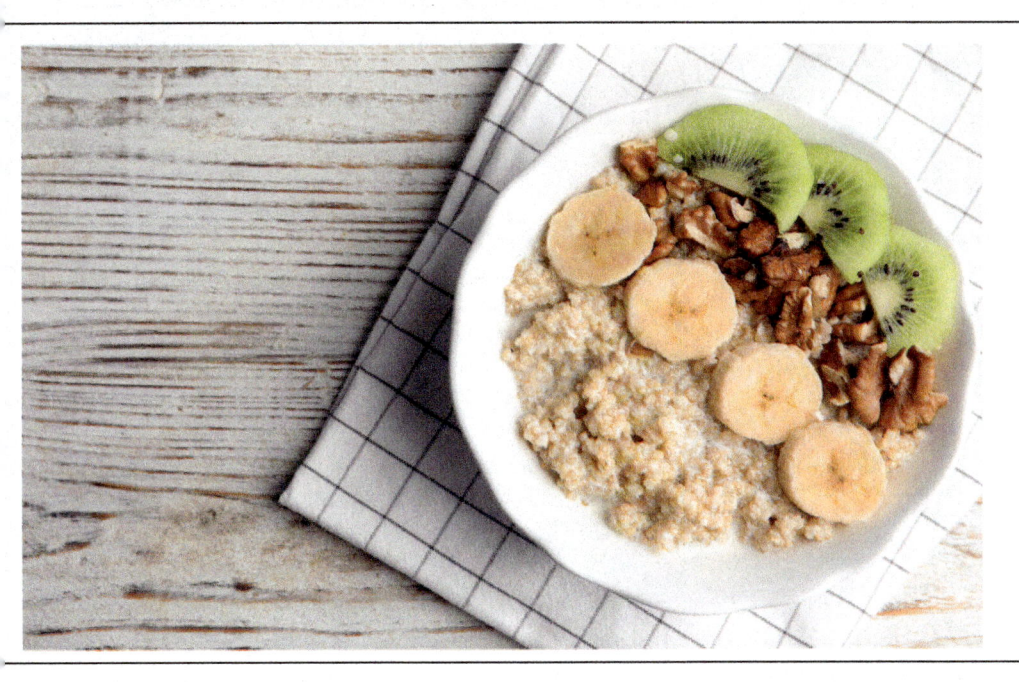

Vibe: A warm and comforting quinoa porridge topped with the freshness of kiwi and a touch of sweetness from maple syrup.

Ingredients

- 1/2 cup quinoa
- 1 cup lactose-free milk
- 1 kiwi, sliced
- Maple syrup for drizzling
- High-quality, very low quantity maple syrup for drizzling
- Unripe banana
- Walnuts

Steps for Cooking:

1. Rinse quinoa thoroughly under cold water.
2. In a saucepan, combine quinoa and lactose-free milk.
3. Bring to a boil, then reduce heat to low, cover, and simmer for about 15 minutes or until quinoa is cooked and the mixture thickens.
4. Serve the quinoa porridge in a bowl.
5. Top with sliced kiwi and drizzle with maple syrup to taste.
6. Enjoy your Low FODMAP quinoa porridge.

TUNA SALAD WITH MIXED GREENS AND A BALSAMIC VINAIGRETTE

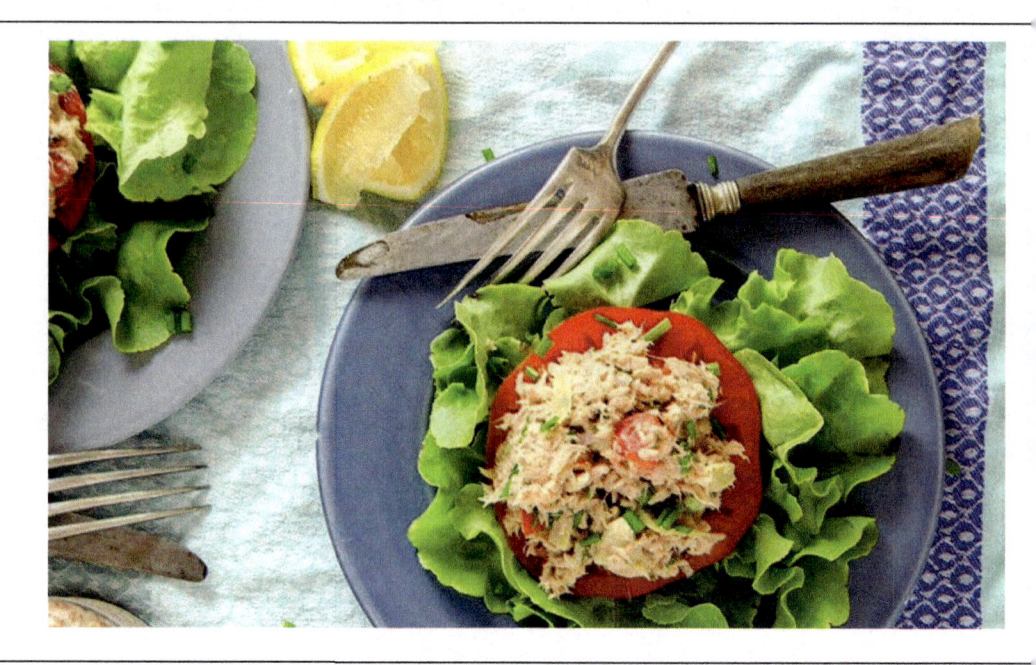

Vibe: A light and nutritious tuna salad with a zesty balsamic vinaigrette.

Ingredients

- 4 oz canned tuna in water, drained
- Mixed greens (e.g., spinach, arugula, lettuce)
- Balsamic vinaigrette (balsamic vinegar, olive oil, salt, and pepper)
- Optional - spring onions (green only) ,

Steps for Cooking:

1. Arrange the mixed greens on a plate.
2. Top with canned tuna.
3. Drizzle with balsamic vinaigrette.
4. Toss to combine and enjoy your Low FODMAP tuna salad.

GRILLED CHICKEN WITH SAUTÉED SPINACH AND ROASTED SWEET POTATOES

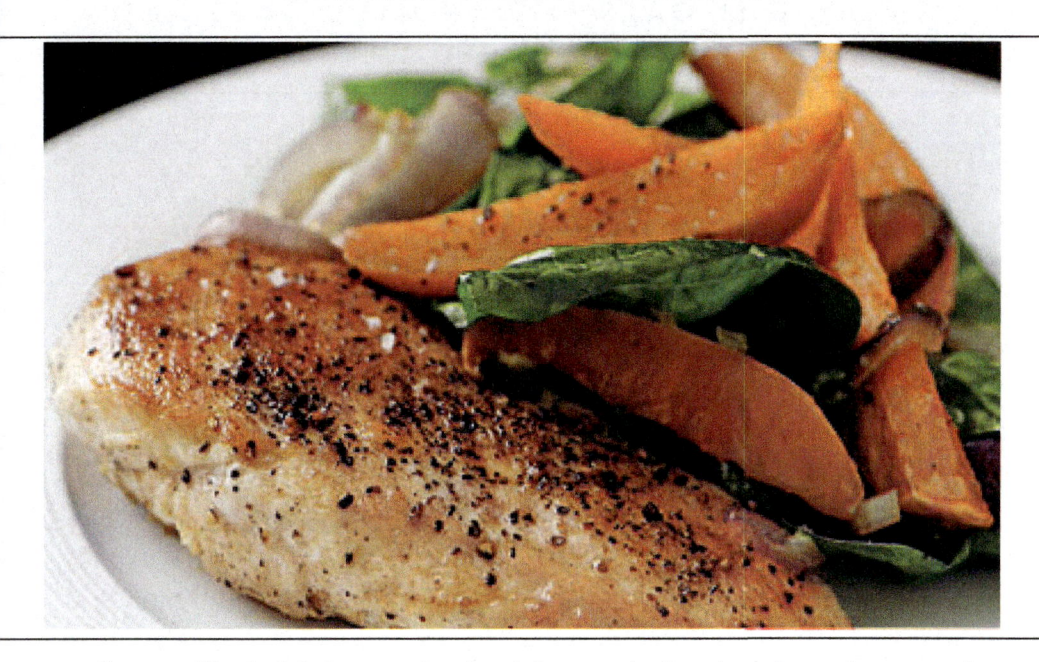

Vibe: Grilled chicken paired with sautéed spinach and roasted sweet potatoes.

Ingredients

- Grilled chicken breast
- Fresh spinach leaves
- less than 70g of Sweet potatoes, roasted
- Olive oil, salt, and pepper for seasoning

Steps for Cooking:

1. Grill chicken breast until cooked to your liking.
2. In a skillet, sauté fresh spinach leaves until wilted.
3. Season with salt and pepper.
4. Roast sweet potatoes until tender and slightly caramelized.
5. Serve grilled chicken with sautéed spinach and roasted sweet potatoes.
6. Enjoy your Low FODMAP grilled chicken with sautéed spinach and sweet potatoes.

DAY 5

OVERNIGHT OATS WITH ROLLED OATS AND LACTOSE-FREE MILK, TOPPED WITH RASPBERRIES

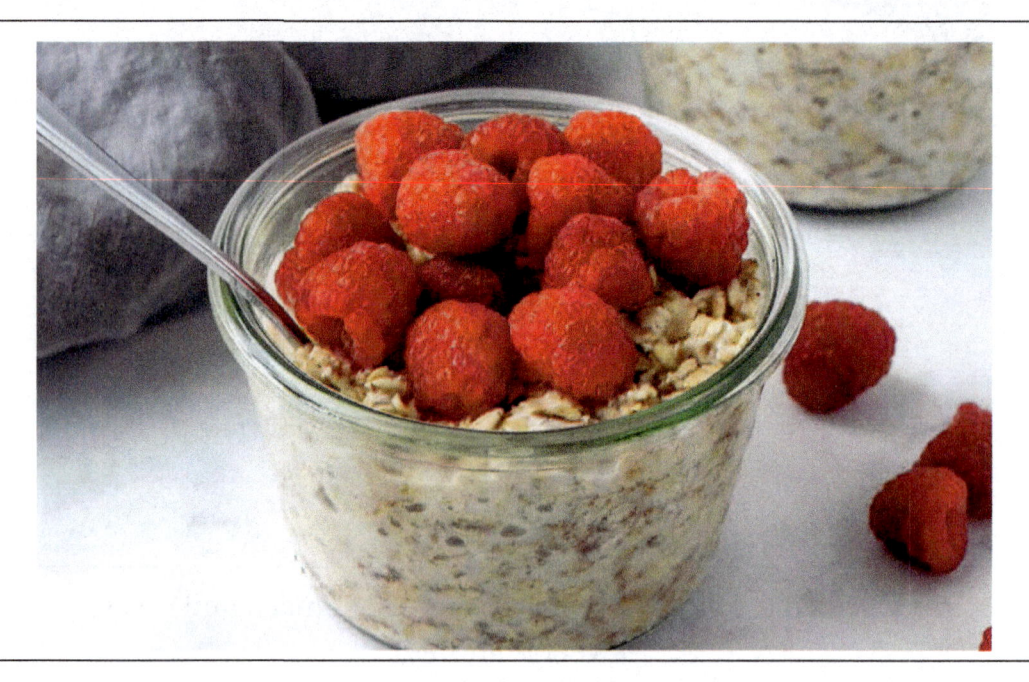

Vibe: A convenient and nutritious breakfast that's ready when you are.

Ingredients

- 1/2 cup rolled oats
- 1 cup lactose-free milk
- 1/2 cup raspberries
- Chia seeds

Steps for Cooking:

1. In a jar or container, combine rolled oats and lactose-free milk.
2. Stir well, cover, and refrigerate overnight.
3. In the morning, give the oats a good stir.
4. Top with fresh raspberries.
5. Enjoy your Low FODMAP overnight oats.

SPINACH AND BACON SALAD WITH A BOILED EGG AND MUSTARD VINAIGRETTE

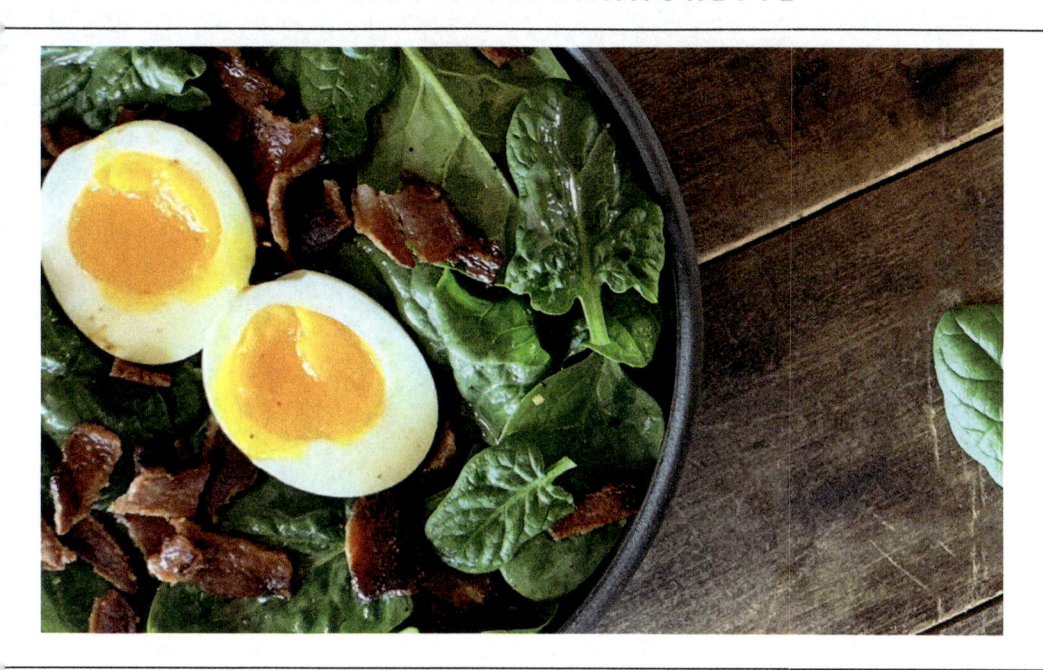

Vibe: A hearty spinach and bacon salad with a boiled egg and tangy mustard vinaigrette.

Ingredients

- Fresh spinach leaves
- Crispy bacon (check for any high FODMAP ingredients)
- 1 boiled egg, sliced
- Mustard vinaigrette (Dijon mustard, olive oil, salt, and pepper)

Steps for Cooking:

1. Arrange fresh spinach leaves on a plate.
2. Top with crispy bacon and sliced boiled egg.
3. Drizzle with mustard vinaigrette.
4. Toss to combine and enjoy your Low FODMAP spinach and bacon salad.

BAKED TURKEY MEATBALLS WITH GLUTEN-FREE PASTA AND A LOW FODMAP MARINARA SAUCE

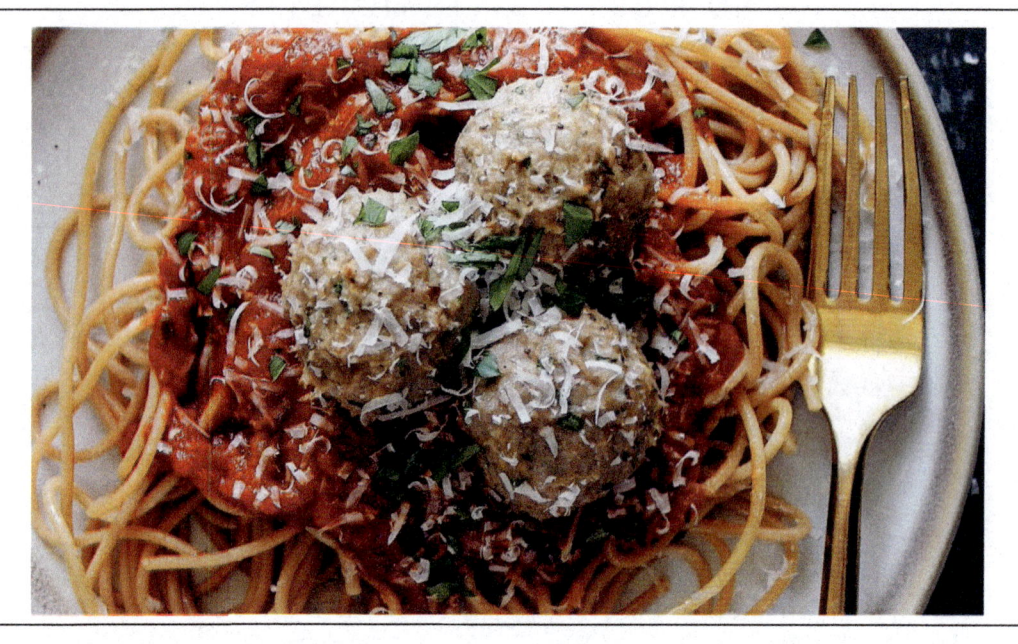

Vibe: A wholesome dinner featuring baked salmon, roasted carrots, and quinoa.

Ingredients

- Turkey meatballs (check for FODMAP content)
- Gluten-free pasta (check for FODMAP content)
- Low FODMAP marinara sauce
- Olive oil, salt, and pepper for seasoning

Steps for Cooking:

1. Preheat the oven to 375°F (190°C).
2. Bake turkey meatballs until cooked through (use a Low FODMAP variety).
3. Cook gluten-free pasta according to package instructions.
4. Heat low FODMAP marinara sauce.
5. Season pasta with olive oil, salt, and pepper.
6. Serve turkey meatballs with gluten-free pasta and marinara sauce.
7. Enjoy your Low FODMAP baked turkey meatballs with gluten-free pasta and marinara sauce.

DAY 6

SPINACH AND FETA CRUSTLESS QUICHE

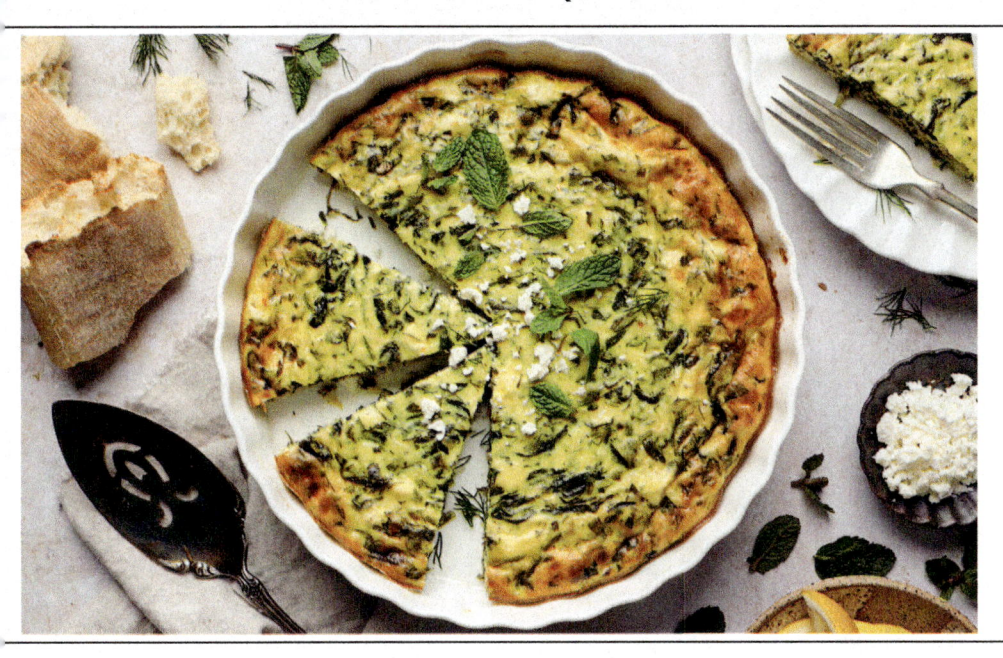

Vibe: A flavorful and satisfying crustless quiche that's easy on the stomach.

Ingredients

- 2 cups fresh spinach leaves
- 1/2 cup crumbled feta cheese
- 6 large eggs
- Salt and pepper to taste
- Olive oil for cooking

Steps for Cooking:

1. Preheat the oven to 350ºF (175ºC).
2. In a skillet, heat a drizzle of olive oil over medium heat.
3. Add fresh spinach leaves and sauté until wilted.
4. In a mixing bowl, whisk the eggs until well beaten.
5. Add crumbled feta cheese, sautéed spinach, salt, and pepper to the eggs. Stir to combine.
6. Grease a pie dish or baking dish.
7. Pour the egg mixture into the dish.
8. Bake for 25-30 minutes or until the quiche is set and lightly browned.
9. Let it cool slightly before slicing.
10. Serve warm and enjoy your Low FODMAP spinach and feta crustless quiche.

CAPRESE SALAD WITH MOZZARELLA, TOMATOES, AND FRESH BASIL

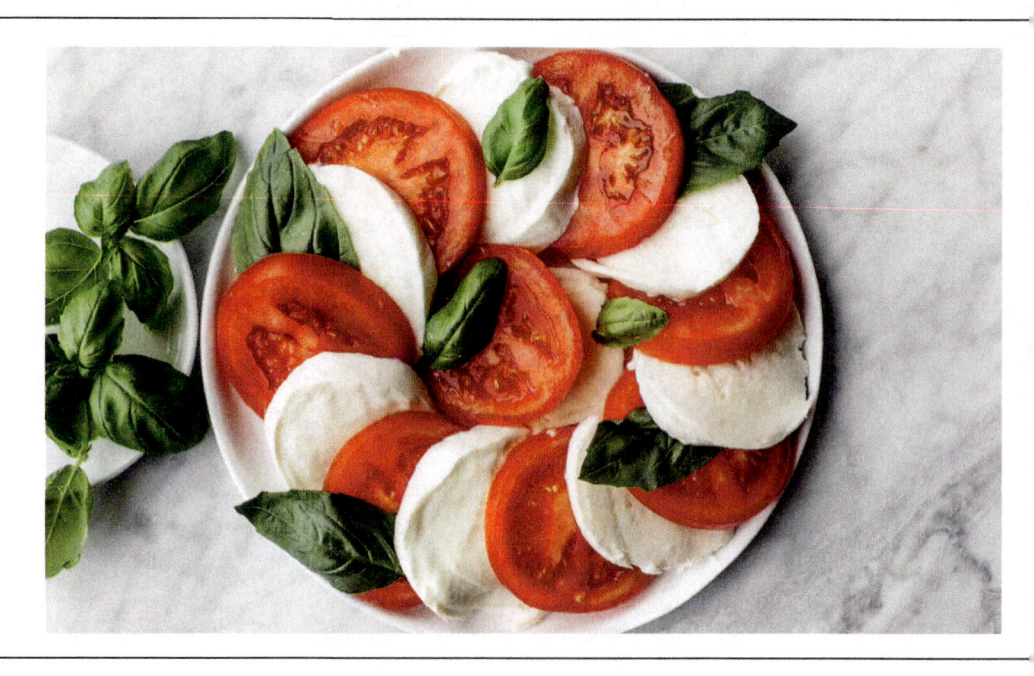

Vibe: A classic and refreshing Caprese salad with a Low FODMAP dressing.

Ingredients

- Fresh mozzarella cheese, sliced
- Ripe tomatoes, sliced
- Fresh basil leaves
- Low FODMAP salad dressing (e.g., olive oil, balsamic vinegar, salt, and pepper)

Steps for Cooking:

1. Arrange mozzarella cheese slices, tomato slices, and fresh basil leaves on a plate.
2. Drizzle with Low FODMAP salad dressing.
3. Season with salt and pepper to taste.
4. Enjoy your Low FODMAP Caprese salad.

PAN-SEARED STEAK WITH MASHED PARSNIPS AND SAUTÉED ZUCCHINI

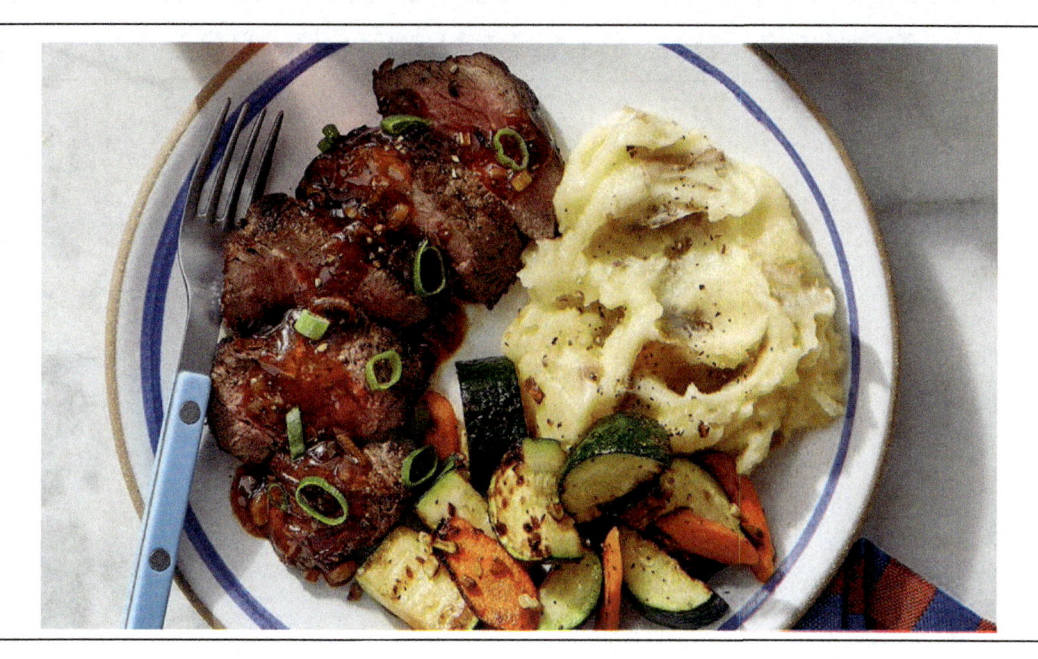

Vibe: A hearty dinner featuring pan-seared steak, creamy mashed parsnips, and sautéed zucchini.

Ingredients

- Steak
- Parsnips, peeled and boiled
- Zucchini, sliced and sautéed
- Olive oil, salt, and pepper for seasoning

Steps for Cooking:

1. Season steak with olive oil, salt, and pepper.
2. Heat a skillet over high heat and sear the steak to your desired level of doneness.
3. Mash boiled parsnips and season with salt and pepper to taste.
4. Sauté sliced zucchini in olive oil until tender.
5. Serve pan-seared steak with mashed parsnips and sautéed zucchini.
6. Enjoy your Low FODMAP pan-seared steak with mashed parsnips and zucchini.

> DAY 7

PEANUT BUTTER AND UNRIPE BANANA TOAST ON GLUTEN-FREE BREAD

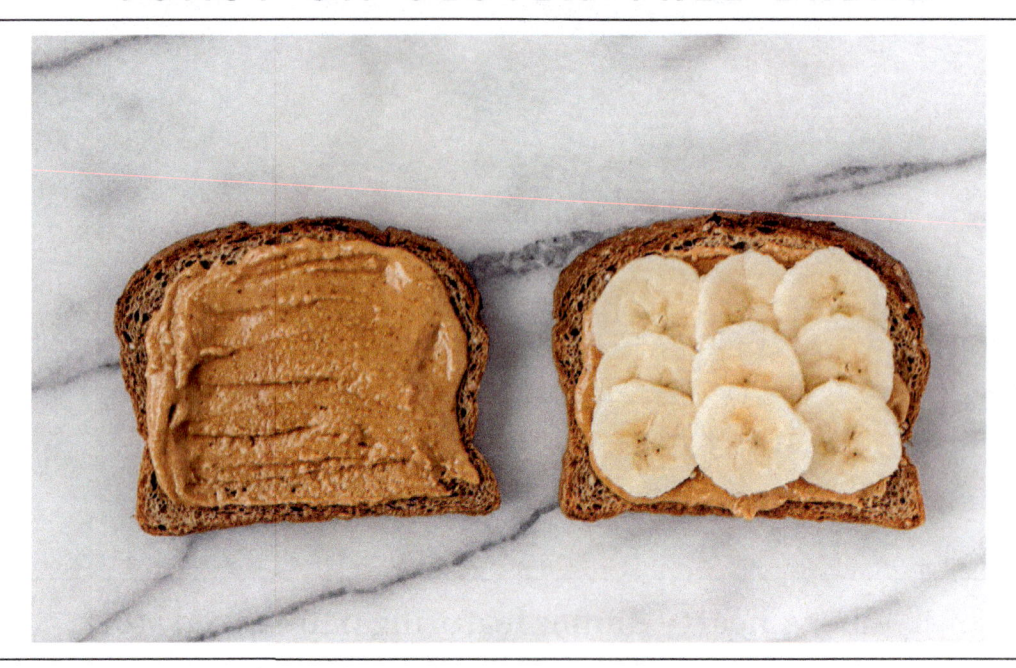

Vibe: A classic combination of peanut butter and banana on gluten-free toast.

Ingredients

- 2 slices of gluten-free bread
- 2 tablespoons peanut butter
- 1 unripe banana, sliced

Steps for Cooking:

1. Toast the gluten-free bread slices.
2. Spread peanut butter evenly on the toasted bread.
3. Arrange sliced unripe banana on top.
4. Press the slices together to make a sandwich, if desired.
5. Enjoy your Low FODMAP peanut butter and banana toast.

SUSHI BOWL WITH COOKED SHRIMP, CUCUMBER, AVOCADO, AND SUSHI RICE

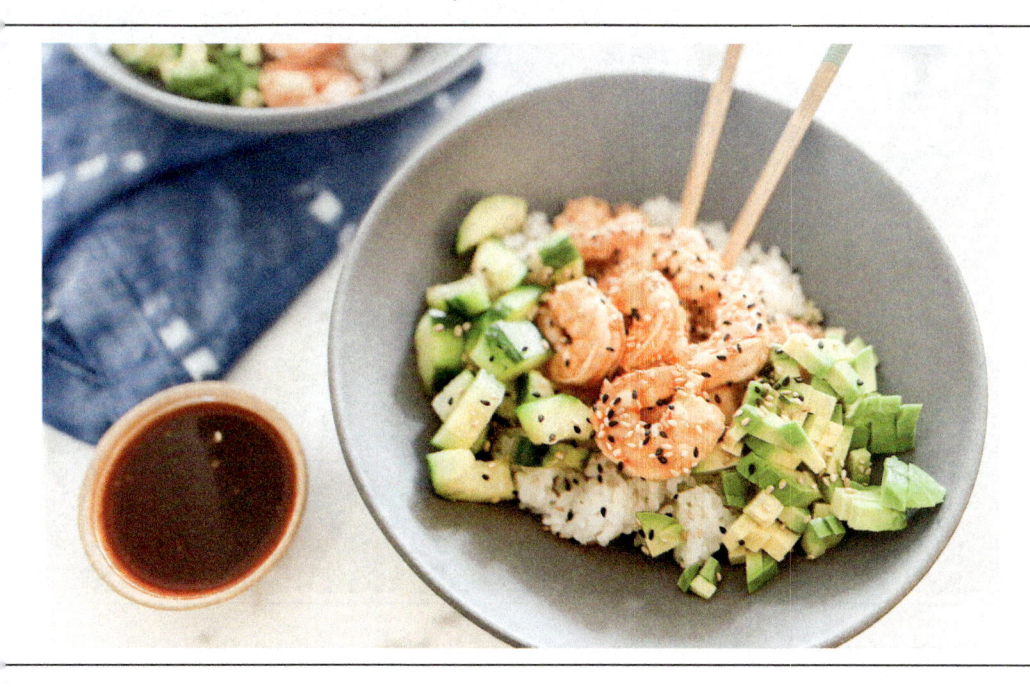

Vibe: A deconstructed sushi experience in a bowl with cooked shrimp, cucumber, avocado, and sushi rice.

Ingredients

- Cooked shrimp
- Sushi rice (check for FODMAP content)
- Sliced cucumber
- Sliced avocado
- Soy sauce (check for FODMAP content)
- Pickled ginger (check for FODMAP content)
- Wasabi (check for FODMAP content)
- Sliced Avocado 30 gram max per serving

Steps for Cooking:

1. In a bowl, layer sushi rice, cooked shrimp, sliced cucumber, and sliced avocado.
2. Drizzle with soy sauce (if tolerated) and garnish with pickled ginger and wasabi.
3. Enjoy your Low FODMAP sushi bowl.

BAKED CHICKEN THIGHS WITH QUINOA AND STEAMED GREEN BEANS

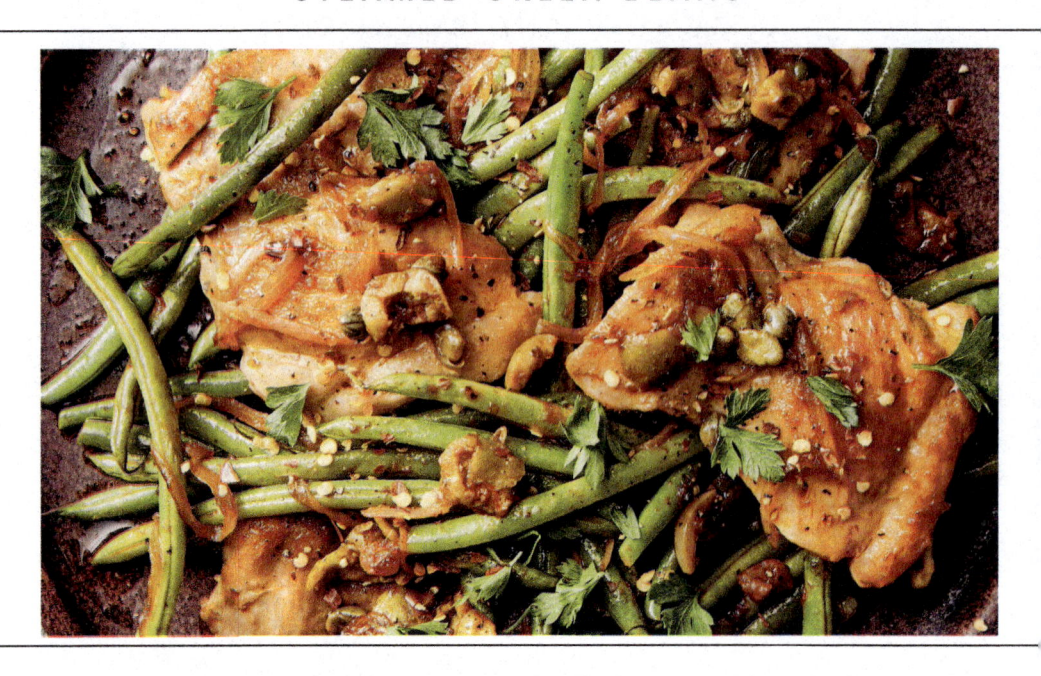

Comforting and nutritious, a perfect blend of juicy chicken, fluffy quinoa, and crisp green beans, creating a wholesome and satisfying meal.

Ingredients

- Chicken thighs
- Quinoa (check for FODMAP content)
- Green beans
- Olive oil, salt, and pepper for seasoning

Steps for Cooking:

1. Preheat the oven to 375°F (190°C).
2. Season chicken thighs with olive oil, salt, and pepper.
3. Bake chicken thighs for about 25-30 minutes or until cooked through.
4. Prepare quinoa according to package instructions (use a Low FODMAP variety).
5. Steam green beans until tender.
6. Serve baked chicken thighs with quinoa and steamed green beans.
7. Enjoy your Low FODMAP baked chicken thighs with quinoa and green beans.

After completing Week 1, it's important to reflect on how your body has responded to the dietary changes. Use the following scale to rate your experiences in various aspects of your health and well-being. Rate each category from 1 to 10 (where 1 is 'no improvement' and 10 is 'significant improvement').

1. Digestive Comfort
- Question: How would you rate the overall comfort of your digestive system this week?
- Rating (1-10): _ _ _ _ _

2. Energy Levels
- Question: How do you feel about your energy levels after following the meal plan for a week?
- Rating (1-10): _ _ _ _ _

3. Sleep Quality
- Question: Have you noticed any changes in the quality of your sleep?
- Rating (1-10): _ _ _ _ _

4. Mood and Mental Clarity
- Question: How has your mood and mental clarity been affected by the dietary changes?
- Rating (1-10): _ _ _ _ _

5. Physical Comfort and Pain Levels
- Question: If you previously experienced any physical discomfort or pain, have you noticed any changes in its intensity or frequency?
- Rating (1-10): _ _ _ _ _

6. Skin Health
- Question: Have there been any noticeable changes in your skin health/appearance?
- Rating (1-10): _ _ _ _ _

7. Cravings and Appetite Control
- Question: How would you rate your control over cravings and appetite this week?
- Rating (1-10): _ _ _ _ _

8. Overall Well-being
- Question: Considering all factors, how would you rate your overall well-being after Week 1?
- Rating (1-10): _ _ _ _ _

FOR SPECIAL *notes*

WEEK 2: WHY FODMAP MATTERS - DEEPENING YOUR UNDERSTANDING

"As you step into Week 2, titled 'Why FODMAP Matters', you'll delve deeper into the connection between FODMAPs and your digestive health. This week is about building upon the foundations laid in Week 1 and beginning to see how specific foods interact with your body. Pay attention to the subtle changes and the way your body responds to this new eating pattern. You're on your way to uncovering the keys to your digestive wellness."

DAY 8

LACTOSE-FREE COTTAGE CHEESE WITH PINEAPPLE CHUNKS

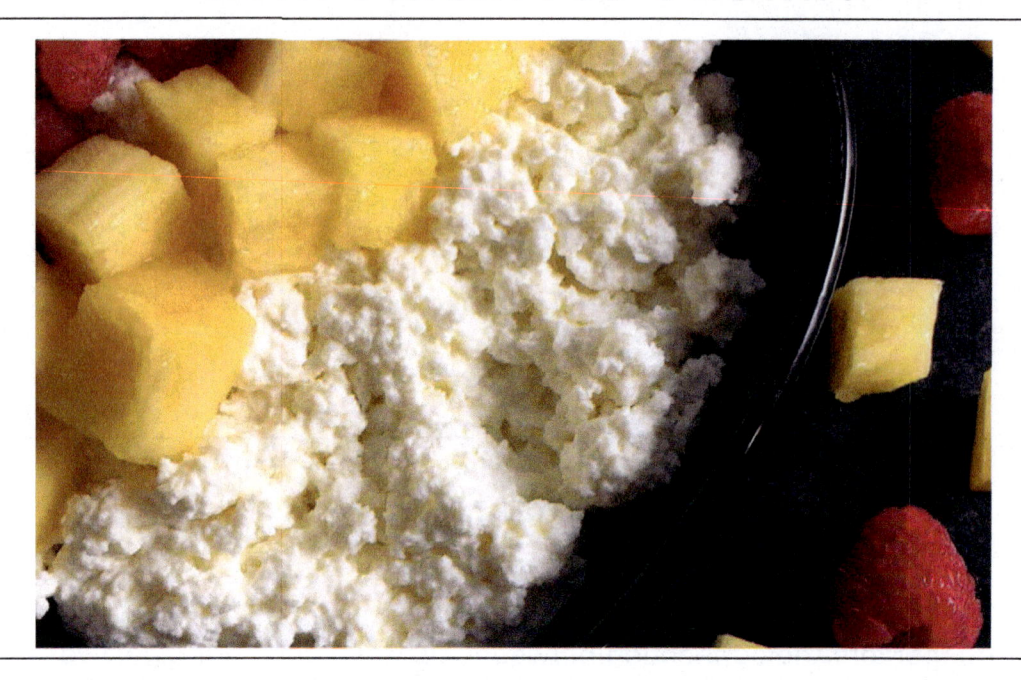

Vibe: A creamy and tropical cottage cheese delight that's easy on the stomach.

Ingredients

- 1 cup lactose-free cottage cheese
- 1/2 cup pineapple chunks

Steps for Cooking:

1. In a bowl, scoop out the lactose-free cottage cheese.
2. Top with pineapple chunks.
3. Stir gently to combine.
4. Enjoy your Low FODMAP cottage cheese with pineapple.

RICE PAPER ROLLS WITH SHRIMP, LETTUCE, CARROTS, AND A DIPPING SAUCE

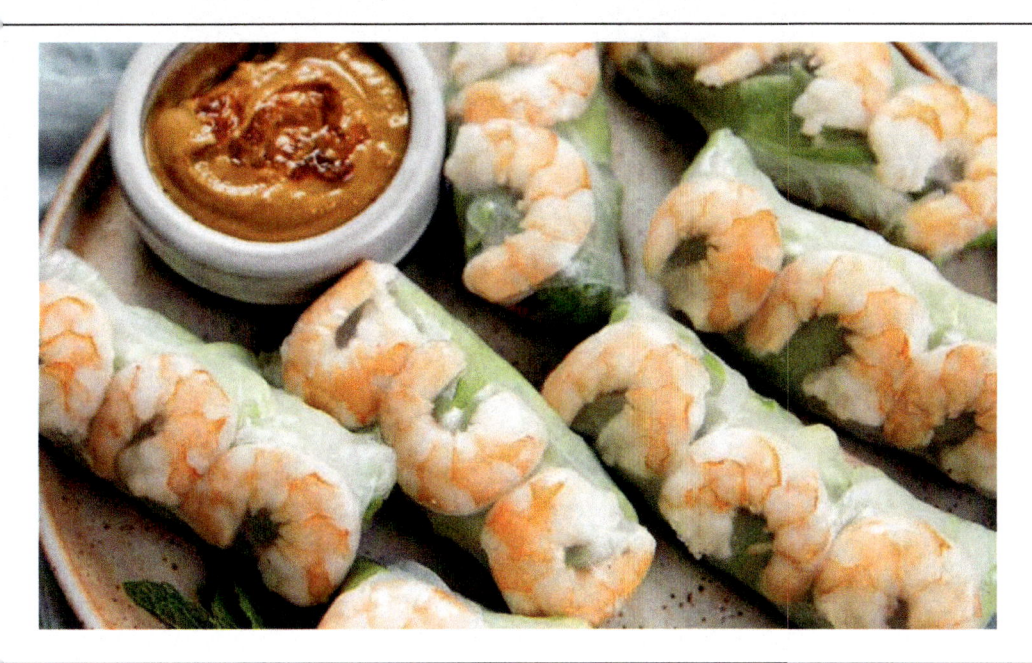

Vibe: Fresh and flavorful rice paper rolls with shrimp and veggies, served with a Low FODMAP dipping sauce.

Ingredients

- Rice paper sheets (check for FODMAP content)
- Cooked shrimp
- Lettuce leaves
- Carrot strips
- Low FODMAP dipping sauce (e.g., a mix of peanut butter, tamari sauce, and a dash of rice vinegar)

Steps for Cooking:

1. Dip a rice paper sheet into warm water to soften it.
2. Lay the softened rice paper on a clean surface.
3. Place cooked shrimp, lettuce leaves, and carrot strips in the center of the rice paper.
4. Roll up the rice paper, folding in the sides, to create a roll.
5. Repeat with the remaining ingredients.
6. Serve with Low FODMAP dipping sauce.
  1. Enjoy your Low FODMAP rice paper rolls.

GRILLED SWORDFISH WITH A SIDE OF SAUTÉED BOK CHOY AND RICE

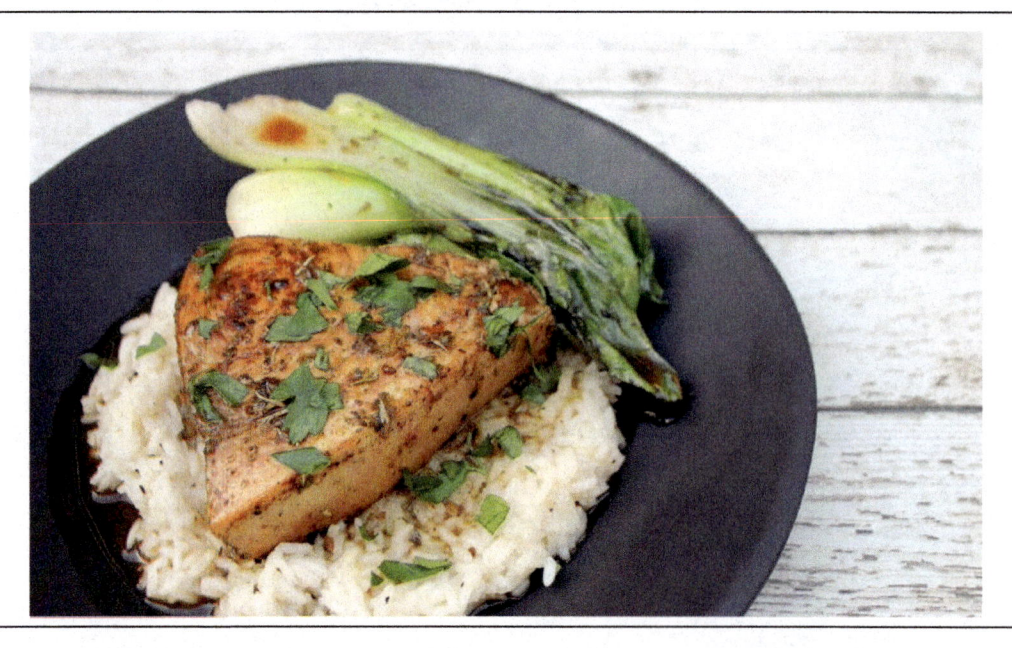

A delightful combination of the ocean's bounty and earth's greens, offering a light yet flavorful experience with perfectly grilled swordfish.

Ingredients

- Swordfish steak
- Bok choy, sautéed
- Rice (check for FODMAP content)
- Olive oil, salt, and pepper for seasoning

Steps for Cooking:

1. Grill swordfish steak until cooked to your liking.
2. Sauté bok choy in olive oil until tender.
3. Season with salt and pepper.
4. Cook rice according to package instructions (use a Low FODMAP variety).
5. Serve grilled swordfish with sautéed bok choy and rice.
6. Enjoy your Low FODMAP grilled swordfish with sautéed bok choy and rice.

DAY 9

SCRAMBLED EGGS WITH SMOKED SALMON AND CHIVES (USE THE GREEN PART)

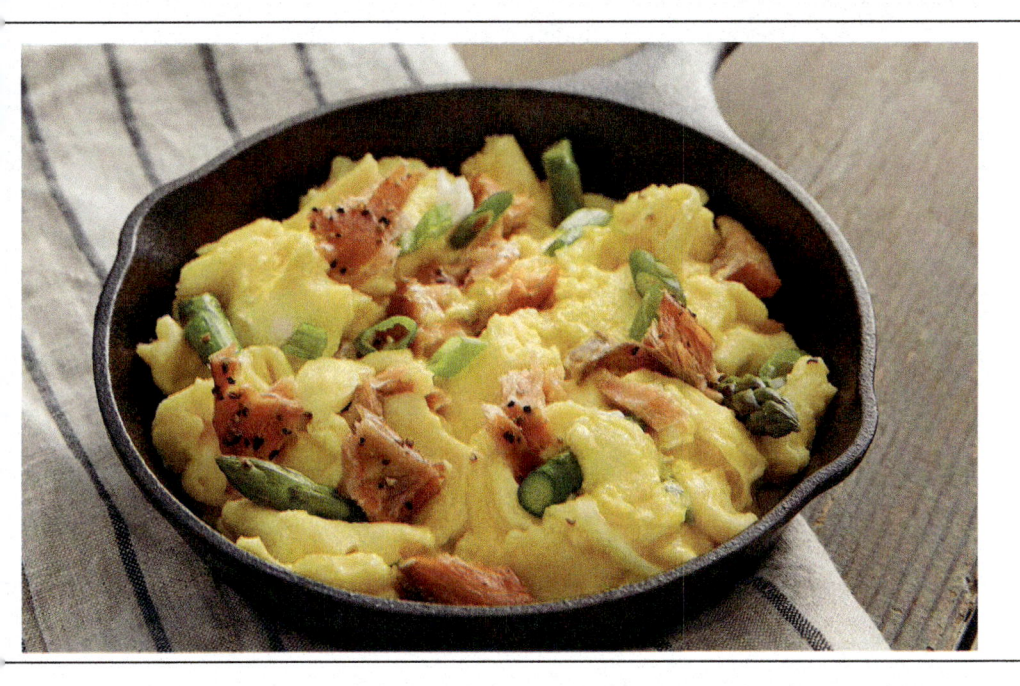

Vibe: A luxurious and savory breakfast with the richness of smoked salmon and a hint of chive freshness.

Ingredients

- 2 large eggs
- 2 oz smoked salmon
- Chives (green part), finely chopped, for garnish
- Salt and pepper to taste
- Olive oil for cooking

Steps for Cooking:

1. In a bowl, whisk the eggs until well beaten.
2. Heat a non-stick skillet over medium heat and add a drizzle of olive oil.
3. Pour the beaten eggs into the skillet.
4. Stir gently as the eggs start to set.
5. When the eggs are almost cooked through, add the smoked salmon.
6. Continue to cook until the eggs are fully set and the salmon is warmed through.
7. Season with salt and pepper to taste.
8. Garnish with chopped chives.
9. Serve hot and savor your Low FODMAP scrambled eggs with smoked salmon.

GRILLED SALMON WITH A SIDE OF GREEN BEANS AND QUINOA

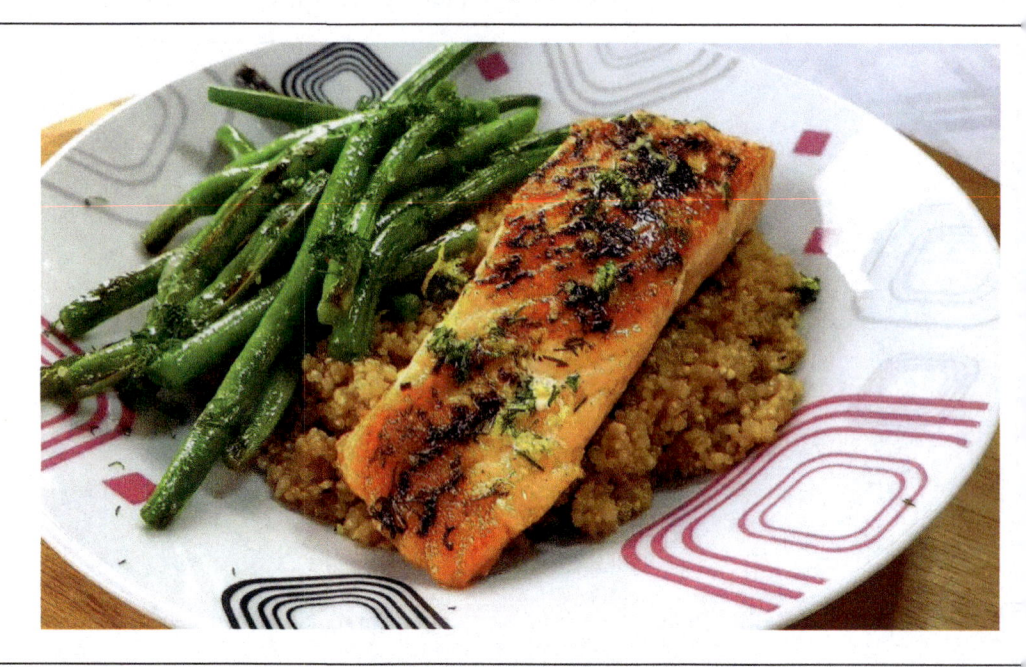

Vibe: A balanced dinner featuring grilled salmon, green beans, and quinoa.

Ingredients

- Grilled salmon fillet
- Green beans, steamed or blanched
- Quinoa (check for FODMAP content)
- Olive oil, salt, and pepper for seasoning

Steps for Cooking:

1. Season the grilled salmon with olive oil, salt, and pepper.
2. Grill the salmon until cooked to your desired level of doneness.
3. Steam or blanch green beans until tender.
4. Prepare quinoa according to package instructions.
5. Serve grilled salmon with a side of green beans and quinoa.
6. Enjoy your Low FODMAP grilled salmon dinner.

PORK AND VEGETABLE KEBABS WITH A SIDE OF POLENTA

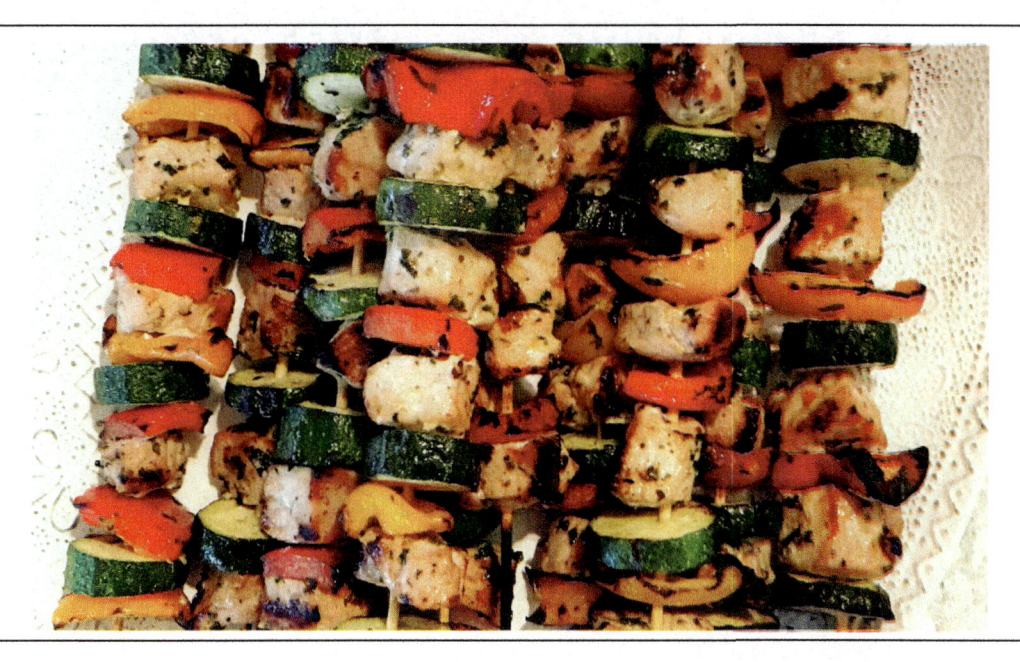

A playful and colorful mix of tender pork and fresh vegetables on a skewer, paired with creamy polenta for a comforting and hearty meal.

Ingredients

- Pork cubes
- Mixed vegetables for kebabs
- Polenta (check for FODMAP content)
- Olive oil, salt, and pepper for seasoning
- Peppers (check for low fodmap amounts)
- Zucchini

Steps for Cooking:

1. Assemble pork and vegetable kebabs.
2. Season with olive oil, salt, and pepper.
3. Grill kebabs until pork is cooked and vegetables are tender.
4. Prepare polenta according to package instructions (use a Low FODMAP variety).
5. Serve pork and vegetable kebabs with a side of polenta.
6. Enjoy your Low FODMAP pork and vegetable kebabs with polenta.

DAY 10

CHIA PUDDING WITH STRAWBERRIES AND A SPRINKLE OF SUNFLOWER SEEDS

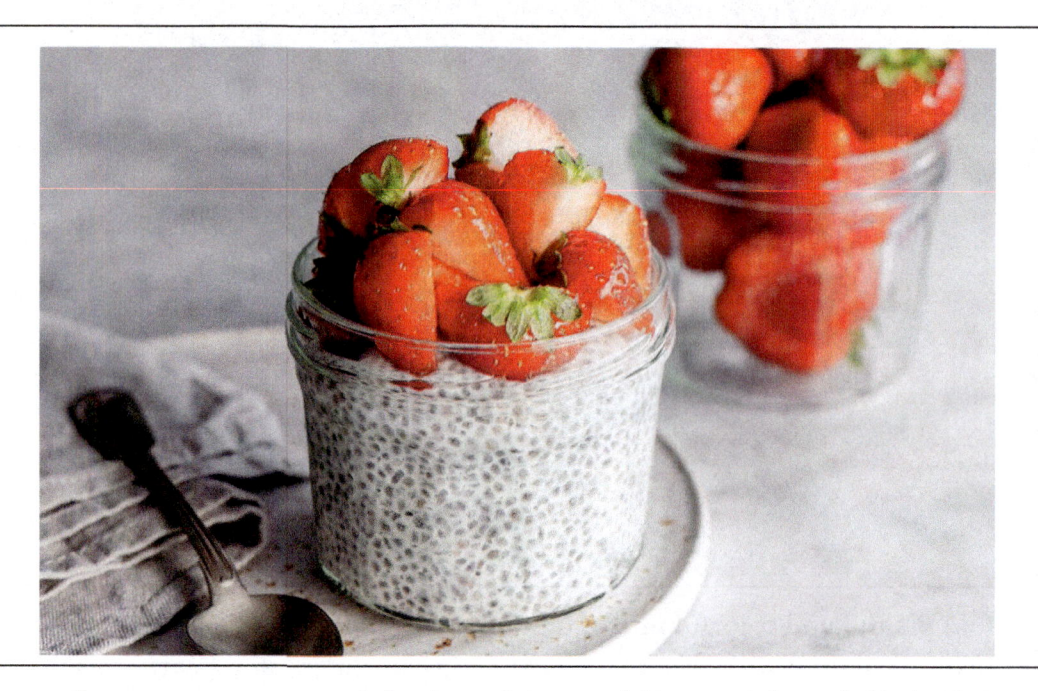

Vibe: A creamy and fruity chia pudding with a delightful crunch of sunflower seeds.

Ingredients

- 2 tablespoons chia seeds
- 1 cup lactose-free milk
- 1/2 cup strawberries, sliced
- Sunflower seeds for sprinkling
- Maple syrup for drizzling (optional for added sweetness)

Steps for Cooking:

1. In a bowl, combine chia seeds and lactose-free milk.
2. Stir well, cover, and refrigerate for at least 2 hours or overnight until the mixture thickens.
3. In the morning, give the chia pudding a good stir.
4. Layer with sliced strawberries.
5. Sprinkle sunflower seeds on top.
6. Drizzle with maple syrup if desired for extra sweetness.
7. Enjoy your Low FODMAP chia pudding with strawberries and sunflower seeds.

SPINACH AND FETA STUFFED CHICKEN BREAST WITH A SIDE SALAD

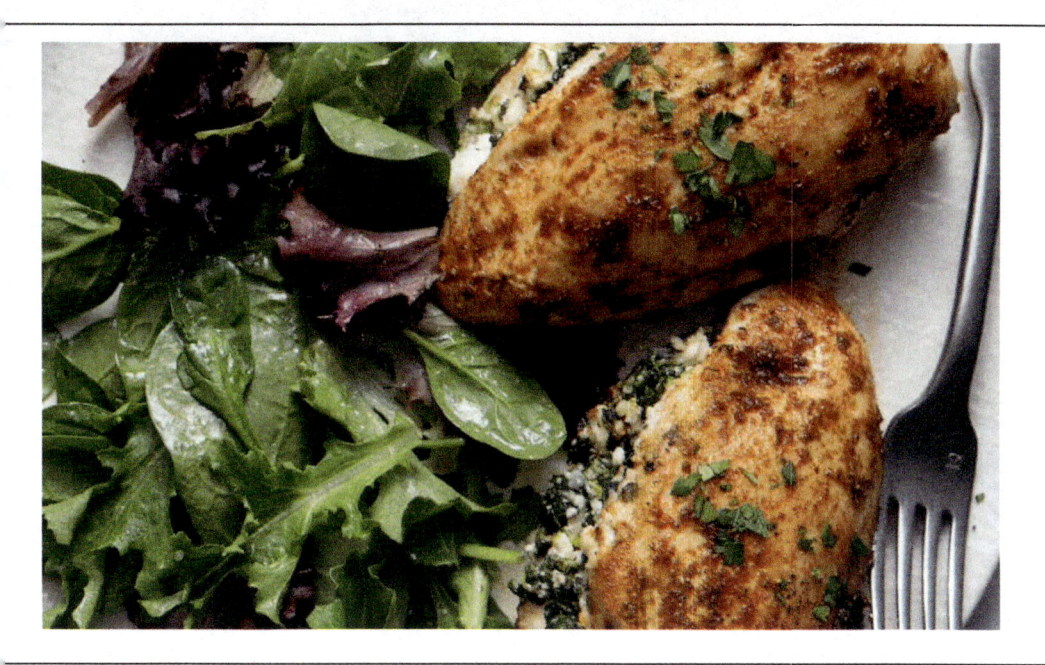

Vibe: A flavorful stuffed chicken breast paired with a refreshing side salad.

Ingredients

- Chicken breast
- Fresh spinach leaves
- Feta cheese (check for FODMAP content)
- Olive oil, salt, and pepper for seasoning
- Side salad with mixed greens (e.g., lettuce, arugula) and a Low FODMAP dressing

Steps for Cooking:

1. Preheat the oven to 375°F (190°C).
2. Cut a pocket into the chicken breast.
3. Stuff the chicken breast with fresh spinach leaves and crumbled feta cheese.
4. Season the chicken breast with olive oil, salt, and pepper.
5. Bake for about 25-30 minutes or until the chicken is cooked through.
6. Serve with a side salad dressed with Low FODMAP dressing.
7. Enjoy your Low FODMAP spinach and feta stuffed chicken breast.

STUFFED BELL PEPPERS WITH GROUND BEEF, RICE, AND TOMATO SAUCE (WITHOUT ONIONS AND GARLIC)

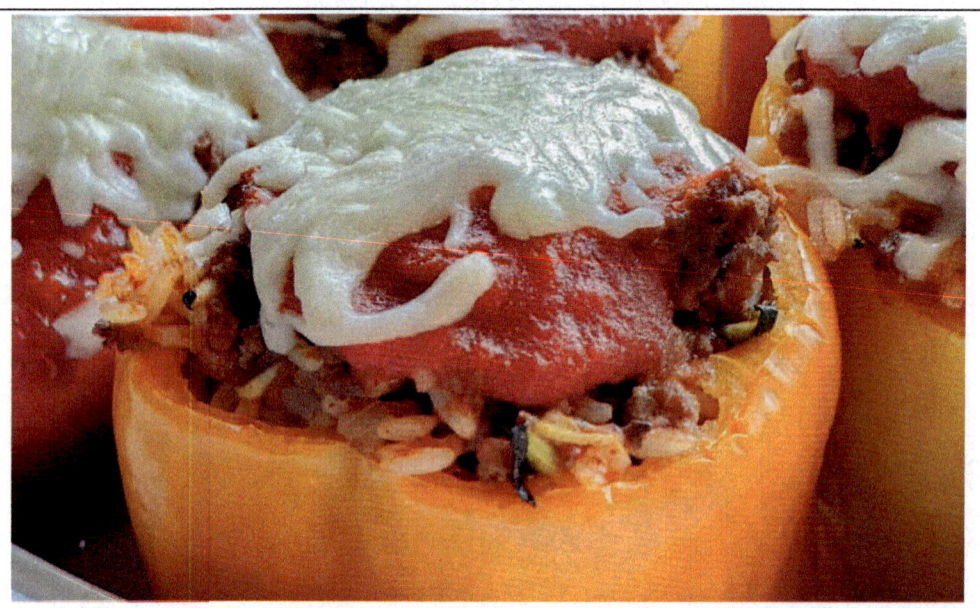

A classic and hearty dish, where bell peppers are lovingly stuffed with savory ground beef and rice, creating a symphony of flavors in each bite.

Ingredients

- Bell peppers
- Ground beef
- Cooked rice (check for FODMAP content)
- Tomato sauce without onions and garlic (check for FODMAP content)
- Olive oil, salt, and pepper for seasoning
- cheese

Steps for Cooking:

1. Preheat the oven to 375°F (190°C).
2. Cut the tops off the bell peppers and remove the seeds.
3. In a skillet, cook ground beef in olive oil until browned.
4. Add cooked rice and tomato sauce (use one without onions and garlic).
5. Season with salt and pepper.
6. Stuff the bell peppers with the ground beef and rice mixture.
7. Place the stuffed bell peppers in a baking dish.
8. Bake for about 25-30 minutes or until the bell peppers are tender.
9. Enjoy your Low FODMAP stuffed bell peppers with ground beef, rice, and tomato sauce.

DAY 11

FODMAP-FRIENDLY GRANOLA WITH LACTOSE-FREE YOGURT AND BLUEBERRIES

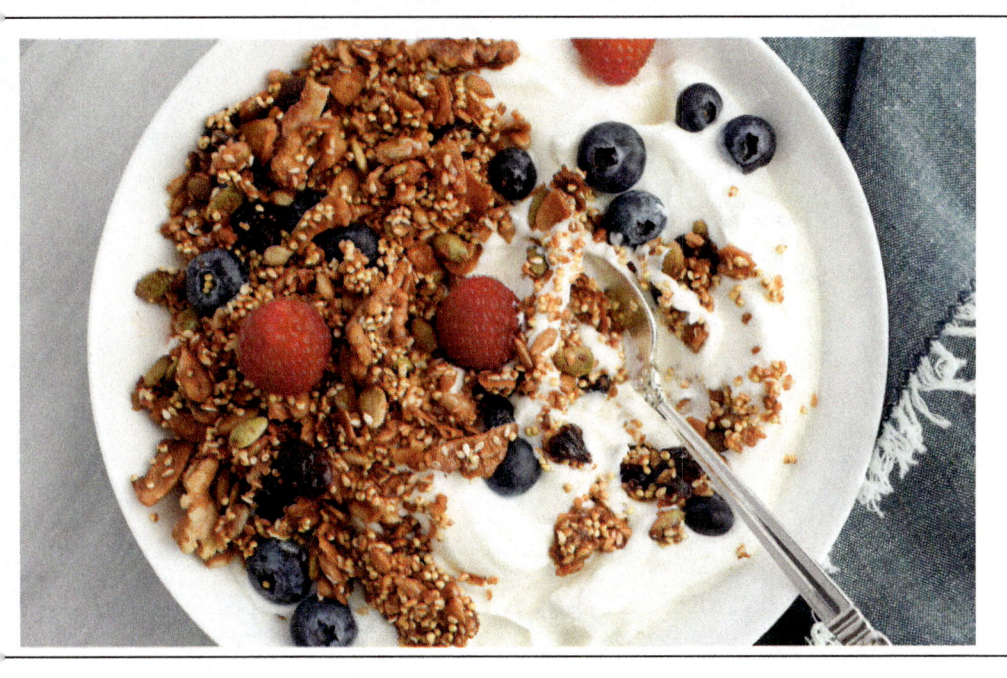

Vibe: A crunchy and wholesome breakfast with the goodness of granola, yogurt, and blueberries.

Ingredients

- 1/2 cup Low FODMAP granola (check label for FODMAP content)
- 1 cup lactose-free yogurt
- 1/2 cup blueberries
- 1-2 raspberries to garnish

Steps for Cooking:

1. In a bowl, scoop out the lactose-free yogurt.
2. Top with Low FODMAP granola.
3. Add fresh blueberries on top.
4. Stir gently to combine if desired.
5. Enjoy your Low FODMAP granola with lactose-free yogurt and blueberries.

CHICKEN AND VEGETABLE STIR-FRY WITH TAMARI SAUCE (NO GARLIC OR ONION)

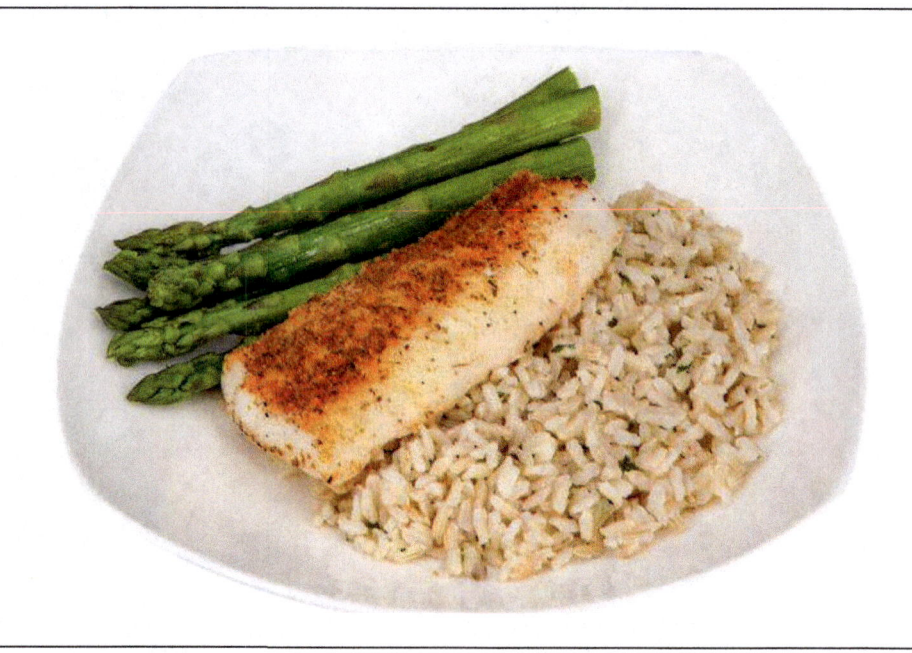

Vibe: A savory and colorful chicken and vegetable stir-fry with a tamari sauce.

Ingredients

- Chicken breast, sliced
- Mixed vegetables (e.g., bell peppers, broccoli, carrots)
- Tamari sauce (check for FODMAP content)
- Olive oil for cooking
- Cooked rice (check for FODMAP content)

Steps for Cooking:

1. Heat a skillet or wok with olive oil over high heat.
2. Add sliced chicken breast and stir-fry until cooked.
3. Remove the chicken from the skillet and set it aside.
4. In the same skillet, stir-fry mixed vegetables until tender.
5. Return the cooked chicken to the skillet.
6. Drizzle with tamari sauce (use a FODMAP-friendly variety).
7. Toss to combine and heat through.
8. Serve over cooked rice.
9. Enjoy your Low FODMAP chicken and vegetable stir-fry.

BAKED CHICKEN BREAST WITH ROASTED POTATOES AND CARROTS

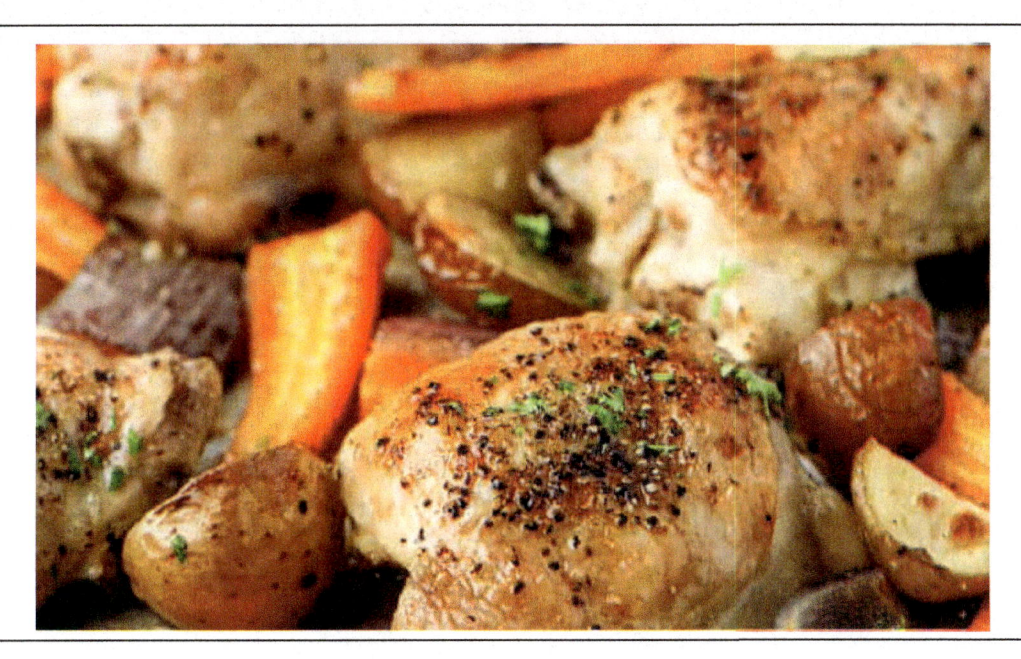

A homely and nourishing meal, combining the simplicity of baked chicken with the rustic charm of roasted potatoes and carrots.

Ingredients

- Chicken breast
- Potatoes (check for FODMAP content)
- Carrots
- Olive oil, salt, and pepper for seasoning

Steps for Cooking:

1. Preheat the oven to 375°F (190°C).
2. Season chicken breast with olive oil, salt, and pepper.
3. Bake chicken breast for about 20-25 minutes or until cooked through.
4. Roast potatoes and carrots until tender and slightly crispy.
5. Serve baked chicken breast with roasted potatoes and carrots.
6. Enjoy your Low FODMAP baked chicken breast with roasted potatoes and carrots.

DAY 12

SPINACH AND BACON FRITTATA

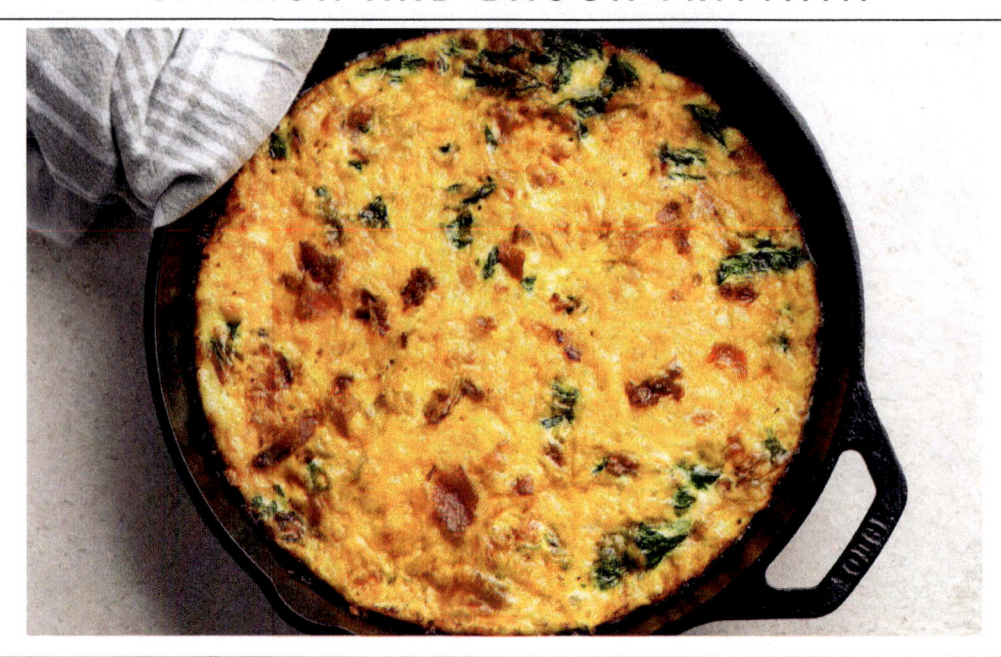

Vibe: A savory and satisfying frittata with the goodness of spinach and bacon.

Ingredients

- 6 large eggs
- 1 cup fresh spinach leaves
- 4 strips of bacon (check for any high FODMAP ingredients)
- Salt and pepper to taste
- Olive oil for cooking

Steps for Cooking:

1. Preheat the oven to 350°F (175°C).
2. In a skillet, cook bacon until crispy, then crumble it. Set aside.
3. In a mixing bowl, whisk the eggs until well beaten.
4. Heat an oven-safe skillet over medium heat with a drizzle of olive oil.
5. Add fresh spinach leaves to the skillet and sauté until wilted.
6. Pour the beaten eggs into the skillet.
7. Sprinkle crumbled bacon evenly over the eggs.
8. Season with salt and pepper to taste.
9. Transfer the skillet to the preheated oven and bake for about 15-20 minutes or until the frittata is set and lightly browned.
10. Slice and serve your Low FODMAP spinach and bacon frittata.

QUINOA BOWL WITH GRILLED ZUCCHINI, EGGPLANT, AND CHERRY TOMATOES

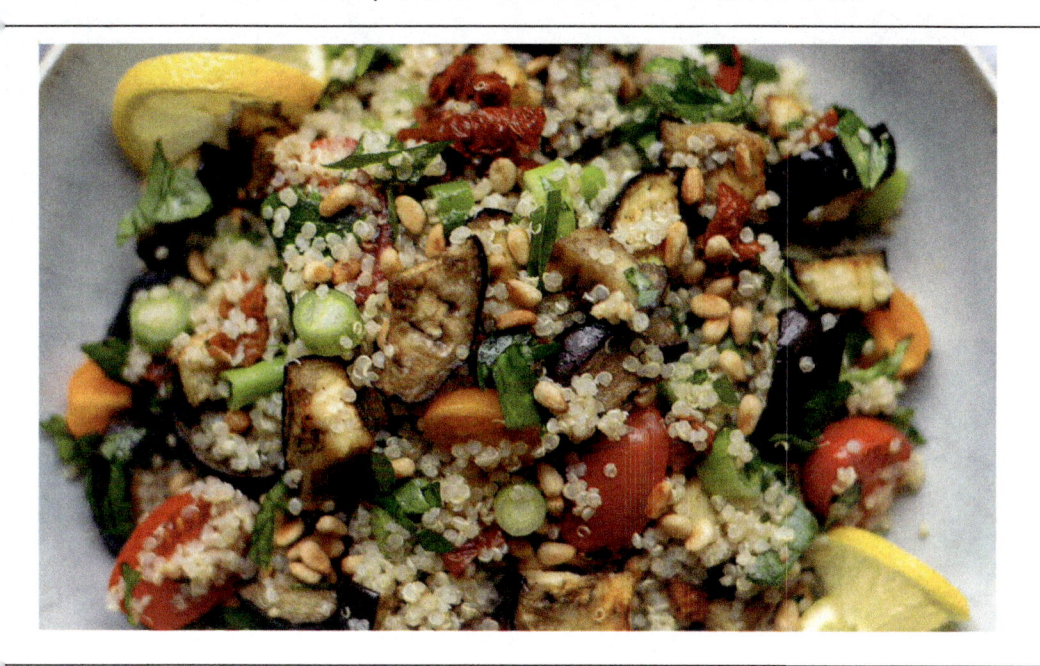

Vibe: A wholesome quinoa bowl with grilled vegetables and cherry tomatoes.

Ingredients

- Cooked quinoa (check for FODMAP content)
- Grilled zucchini slices
- Grilled eggplant slices
- Cherry tomatoes
- Olive oil, salt, and pepper for seasoning

Steps for Cooking:

1. Prepare cooked quinoa according to package instructions.
2. Grill zucchini slices and eggplant slices until tender.
3. Halve cherry tomatoes.
4. In a bowl, combine cooked quinoa, grilled zucchini, grilled eggplant, and cherry tomatoes.
5. Drizzle with olive oil and season with salt and pepper.
6. Toss to combine and enjoy your Low FODMAP quinoa bowl.

GRILLED TURKEY BURGERS ON GLUTEN-FREE BUNS WITH LETTUCE AND TOMATO

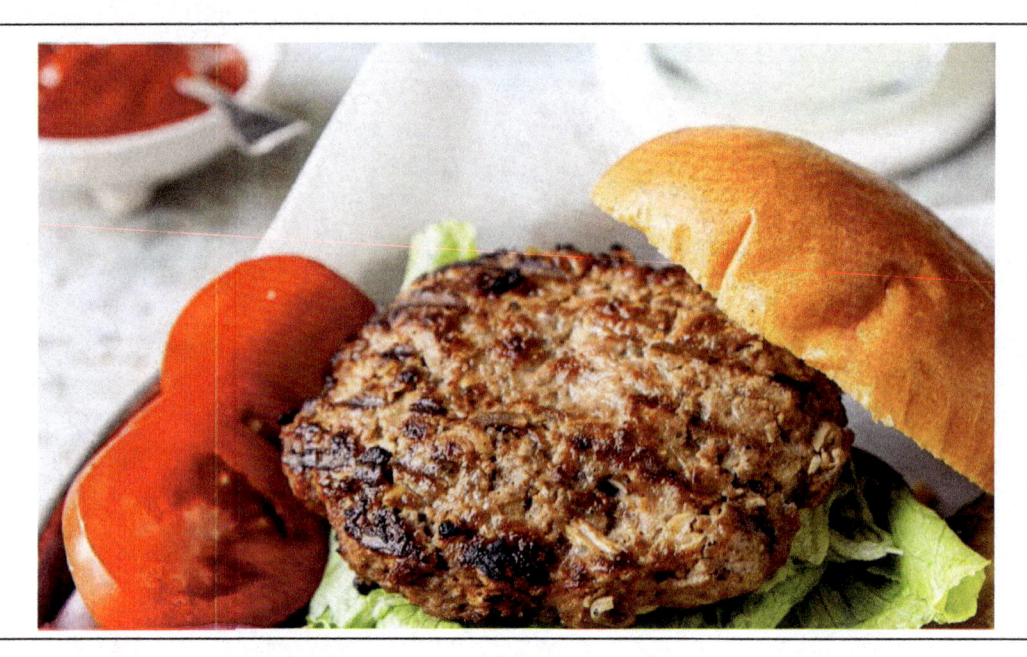

A lighter take on the classic burger, offering a succulent turkey patty on a gluten-free bun, perfect for a guilt-free indulgence.

Ingredients

- Turkey burger patties
- Gluten-free burger buns (check for FODMAP content)
- Lettuce leaves
- Sliced tomatoes
- Olive oil, salt, and pepper for seasoning

Steps for Cooking:

1. Preheat the grill or a skillet over medium-high heat.
2. Season turkey burger patties with olive oil, salt, and pepper.
3. Grill the turkey burgers until cooked through.
4. Toast gluten-free burger buns on the grill or in a toaster.
5. Assemble the burgers with lettuce leaves and sliced tomatoes.
6. Serve your Low FODMAP grilled turkey burgers on gluten-free buns.
7. Enjoy your burger with a side of your choice.

DAY 13

SMOOTHIE BOWL TOPPED WITH SLICED KIWI, SHREDDED COCONUT, AND WALNUTS

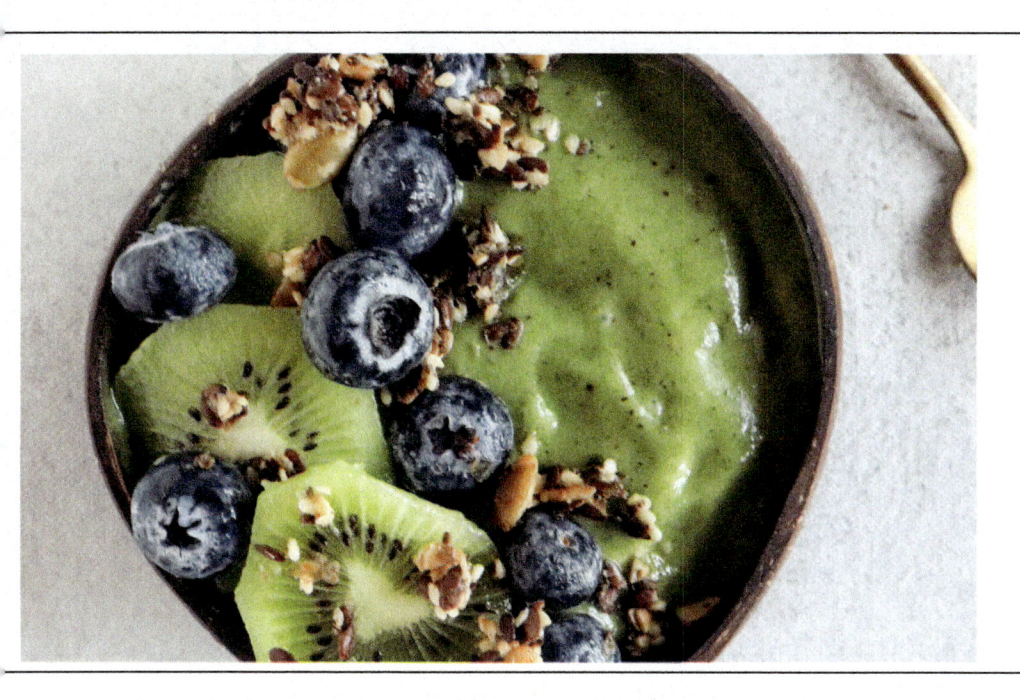

Vibe: A classic combination of peanut butter and banana on gluten-free toast.

Ingredients

- 1/2 cup lactose-free yogurt
- 1/2 banana (unripe)
- 1/2 cup frozen strawberries
- 1/4 cup shredded coconut
- 1/4 cup sliced Walnuts
- 1 kiwi, sliced

Steps for Cooking:

1. In a blender, combine lactose-free yogurt, unripe banana, and frozen strawberries.
2. Blend until smooth and creamy.
3. Pour the smoothie into a bowl.
4. Top with sliced kiwi, shredded coconut, and sliced almonds.
5. Enjoy your Low FODMAP smoothie bowl.

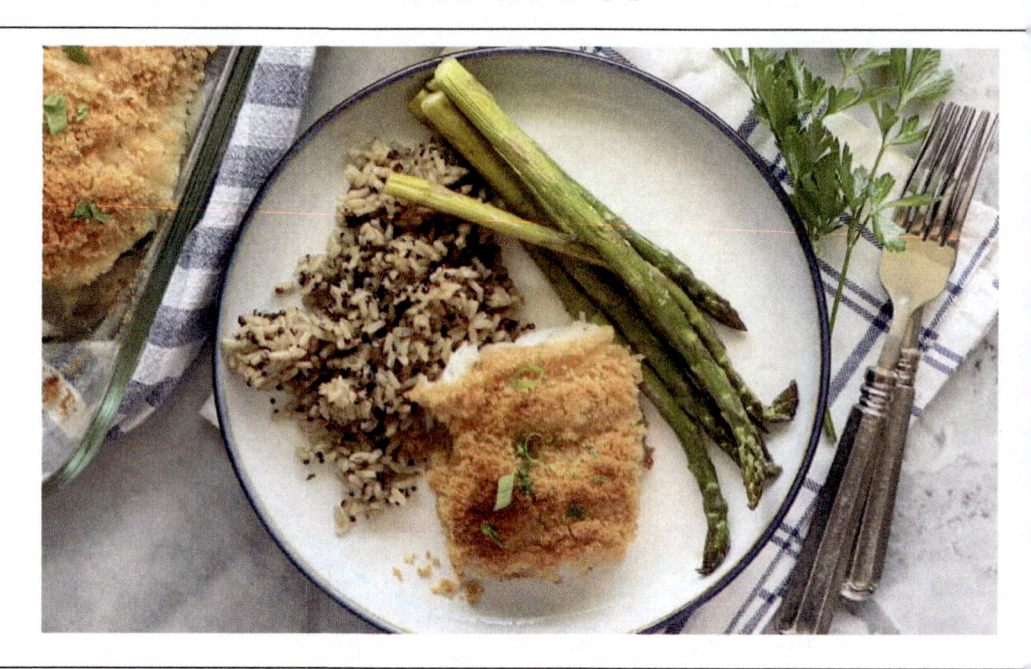

BAKED COD WITH STEAMED ASPARAGUS AND BROWN RICE

Vibe: A light and nutritious dinner featuring baked cod, steamed asparagus, and brown rice.

Ingredients

- Cod fillet
- Asparagus spears, steamed
- Brown rice (check for FODMAP content)
- Lemon wedges
- Olive oil, salt, and pepper for seasoning

Steps for Cooking:

1. Preheat the oven to 375°F (190°C).
2. Season the cod fillet with olive oil, salt, and pepper.
3. Bake the cod fillet for about 15-20 minutes or until it flakes easily with a fork.
4. Serve the baked cod with steamed asparagus and brown rice.
5. Garnish with lemon wedges.
6. Enjoy your Low FODMAP baked cod dinner.

LEMON AND HERB ROASTED CHICKEN WITH STEAMED BROCCOLI AND QUINOA

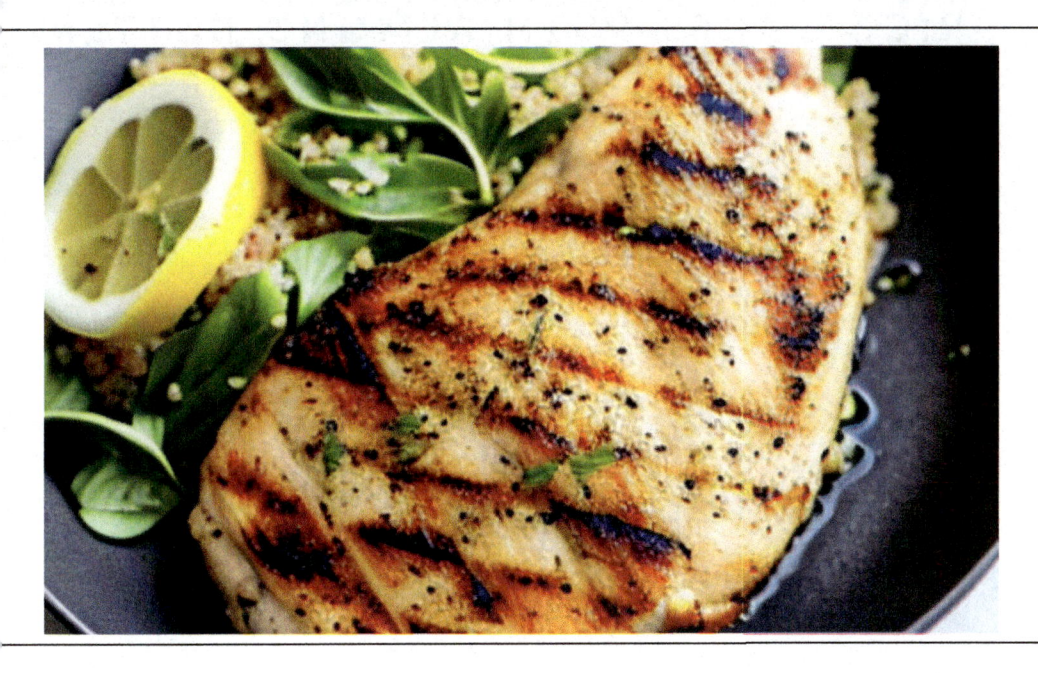

A zesty and refreshing meal, where lemon and herbs bring the chicken to life, accompanied by the wholesomeness of steamed broccoli and quinoa.

Ingredients

- Chicken pieces (e.g., thighs, drumsticks)
- Lemon juice
- Fresh herbs (e.g., rosemary, thyme)
- Broccoli florets
- Quinoa (check for FODMAP content)
- Olive oil, salt, and pepper for seasoning

Steps for Cooking:

1. Preheat the oven to 375°F (190°C).
2. Marinate chicken pieces with lemon juice, fresh herbs, olive oil, salt, and pepper.
3. Roast the chicken until cooked through and golden brown.
4. Steam broccoli florets until tender.
5. Prepare quinoa according to package instructions (use a Low FODMAP variety).
6. Serve lemon and herb-roasted chicken with steamed broccoli and quinoa.
7. Enjoy your Low FODMAP lemon and herb-roasted chicken with broccoli and quinoa.

DAY 14

RICE CAKES WITH ALMOND BUTTER AND SLICED STRAWBERRIES

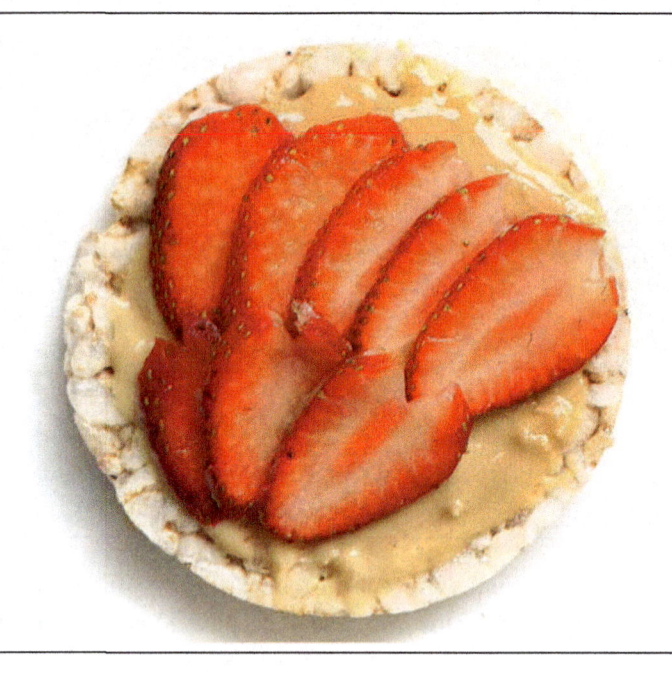

Vibe: A quick and crunchy breakfast with the creaminess of almond butter and the freshness of strawberries.

Ingredients

- 2 rice cakes
- 2 tablespoons almond butter
- 1/2 cup sliced strawberries

Steps for Cooking:

1. Spread almond butter evenly on each rice cake.
2. Top with sliced strawberries.
3. Enjoy your Low FODMAP rice cakes with almond butter and strawberries.

TURKEY AND CHEDDAR CHEESE QUESADILLA ON CORN TORTILLAS

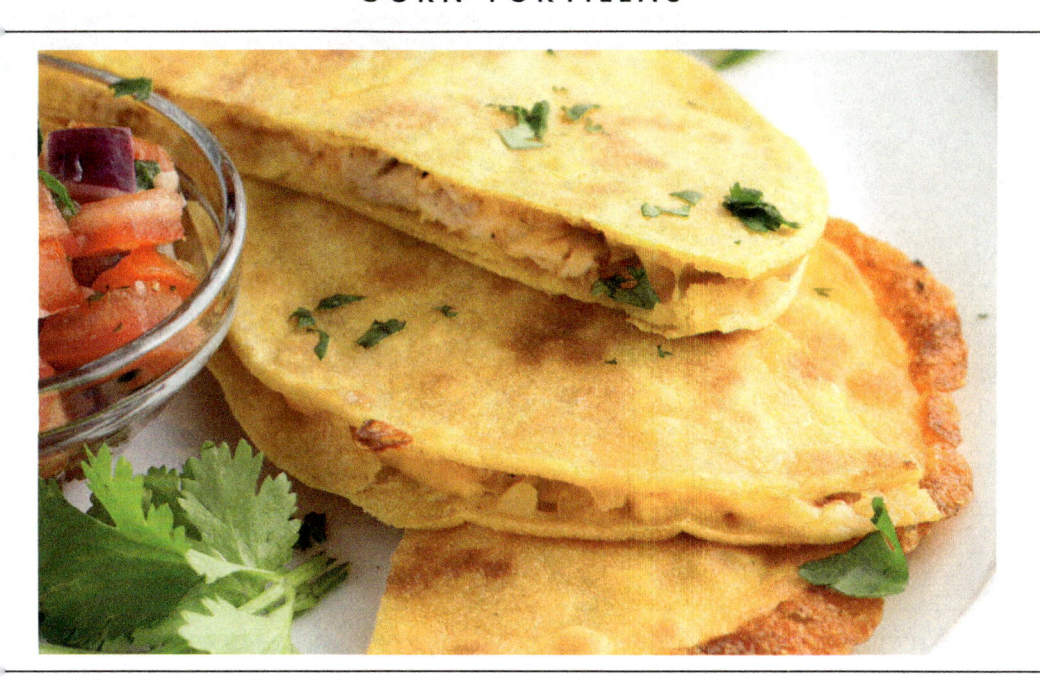

Vibe: A cheesy and satisfying turkey and cheddar cheese quesadilla.

Ingredients

- Slices of turkey
- Slices of cheddar cheese (check for FODMAP content)
- Corn tortillas
- Olive oil for cooking
- Sliced bell peppers (optional for added flavor)

Steps for Cooking:

1. Lay out a corn tortilla.
2. Place slices of turkey, cheddar cheese, and optional bell peppers on half of the tortilla.
3. Fold the tortilla in half to create a quesadilla.
4. Heat a skillet with olive oil over medium heat.
5. Cook the quesadilla until it's golden brown on both sides.
6. Slice and serve.
7. Enjoy your Low FODMAP turkey and cheddar cheese quesadilla.

SEARED TUNA WITH A SESAME SEED CRUST AND A SIDE OF SAUTÉED SPINACH

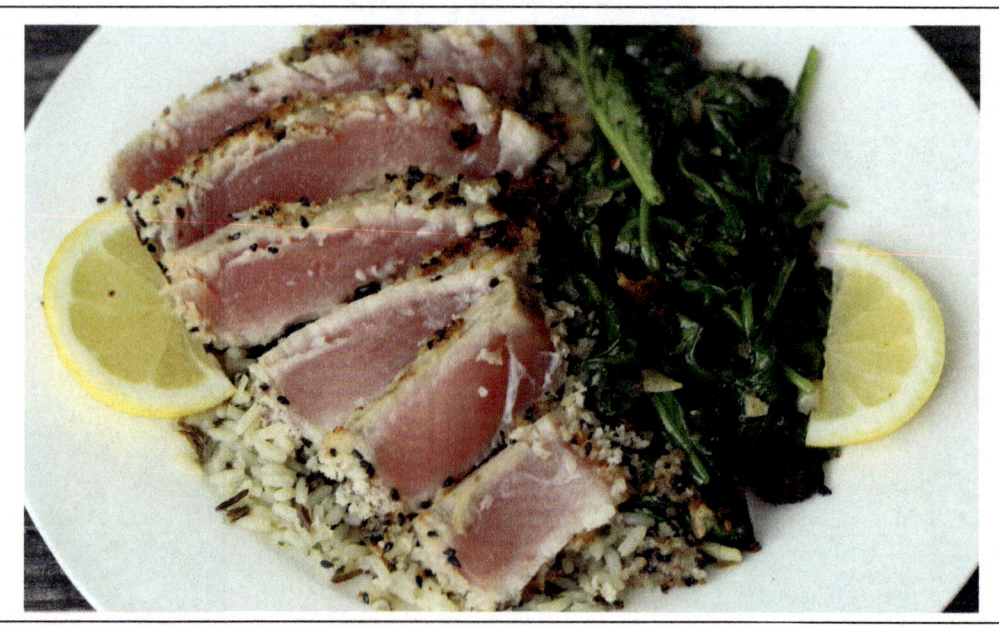

An elegant and sophisticated dish, showcasing a beautifully seared tuna with a crunchy sesame crust, paired with delicately sautéed spinach.

Ingredients

- Tuna steaks
- Sesame seeds
- Fresh spinach leaves
- Olive oil, salt, and pepper for seasoning

Steps for Cooking:

1. Coat tuna steaks with sesame seeds, pressing them onto the surface.
2. Heat a skillet over high heat and sear tuna steaks until rare to medium-rare.
3. In a separate skillet, sauté fresh spinach leaves in olive oil until wilted.
4. Season spinach with salt and pepper.
5. Serve seared tuna with sautéed spinach.
6. Enjoy your Low FODMAP seared tuna with sesame seed crust and sautéed spinach.

After completing Week 2, it's important to reflect on how your body has responded to the dietary changes. Use the following scale to rate your experiences in various aspects of your health and well-being. Rate each category from 1 to 10 (where 1 is 'no improvement' and 10 is 'significant improvement').

1. Digestive Comfort
- Question: How would you rate the overall comfort of your digestive system this week?
- Rating (1-10): _ _ _ _ _

2. Energy Levels
- Question: How do you feel about your energy levels after following the meal plan for a week?
- Rating (1-10): _ _ _ _ _

3. Sleep Quality
- Question: Have you noticed any changes in the quality of your sleep?
- Rating (1-10): _ _ _ _ _

4. Mood and Mental Clarity
- Question: How has your mood and mental clarity been affected by the dietary changes?
- Rating (1-10): _ _ _ _ _

5. Physical Comfort and Pain Levels
- Question: If you previously experienced any physical discomfort or pain, have you noticed any changes in its intensity or frequency?
- Rating (1-10): _ _ _ _ _

6. Skin Health
- Question: Have there been any noticeable changes in your skin health/appearance?
- Rating (1-10): _ _ _ _ _

7. Cravings and Appetite Control
- Question: How would you rate your control over cravings and appetite this week?
- Rating (1-10): _ _ _ _ _

8. Overall Well-being
- Question: Considering all factors, how would you rate your overall well-being after Week 1?
- Rating (1-10): _ _ _ _ _

FOR SPECIAL
notes

WEEK 3: DECODING THE DIGESTIVE DILEMMA - IDENTIFYING YOUR TRIGGERS

"Welcome to Week 3, 'Decoding the Digestive Dilemma'. This crucial week focuses on identifying your unique triggers and understanding the symptoms associated with FODMAP sensitivities. You're now at the heart of your journey, making pivotal discoveries about how your body reacts to different foods. Embrace this week as an opportunity for significant learning and personal growth in your quest for better gut health."

DAY 15

VEGETABLE AND BACON BREAKFAST BURRITO WITH CORN TORTILLAS

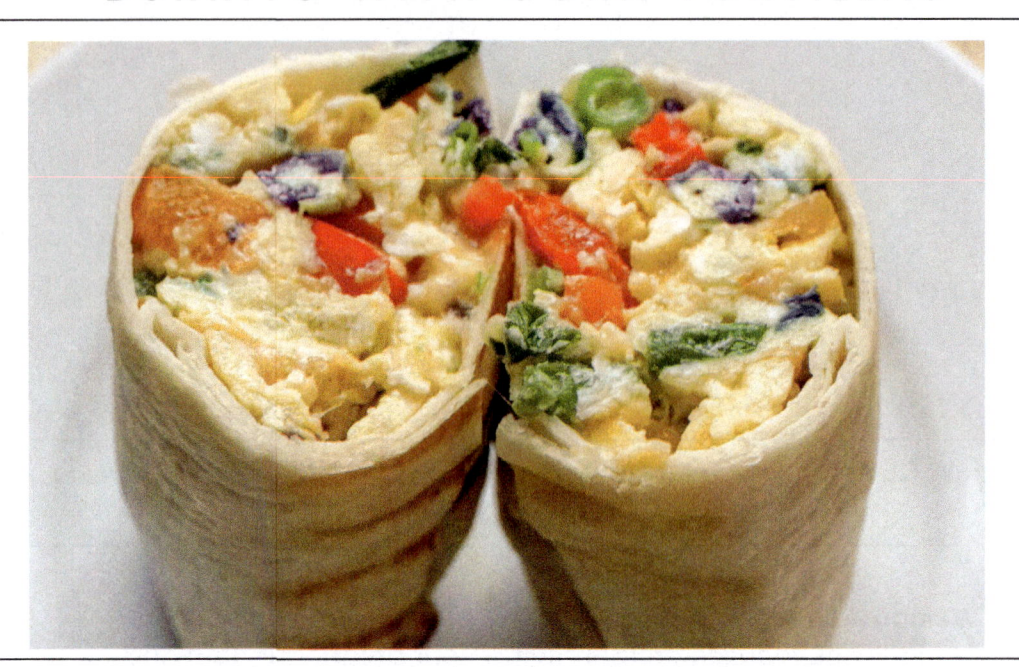

Vibe: A hearty and flavorful breakfast burrito with a Low FODMAP twist.

Ingredients

- 2 corn tortillas
- 4 strips of bacon (check for any high FODMAP ingredients)
- 1/2 cup scrambled eggs
- 1/4 cup diced red bell peppers
- 1/4 cup diced tomatoes (remove seeds)
- Salt and pepper to taste
- Spring onions and mixed leaves

Steps for Cooking:

1. Cook bacon until crispy, then crumble it. Set aside.
2. In a skillet, sauté diced red bell peppers until slightly softened.
3. Add diced tomatoes and cook briefly.
4. Add scrambled eggs to the skillet and cook until set.
5. Warm corn tortillas in a dry skillet or microwave.
6. Fill each tortilla with the scrambled egg mixture and crumbled bacon.
7. Season with salt and pepper to taste.
8. Roll up the tortillas to create breakfast burritos.
9. Serve warm and enjoy your Low FODMAP vegetable and bacon breakfast burrito.

ZUCCHINI NOODLES WITH GRILLED SHRIMP AND PESTO (WITHOUT GARLIC)

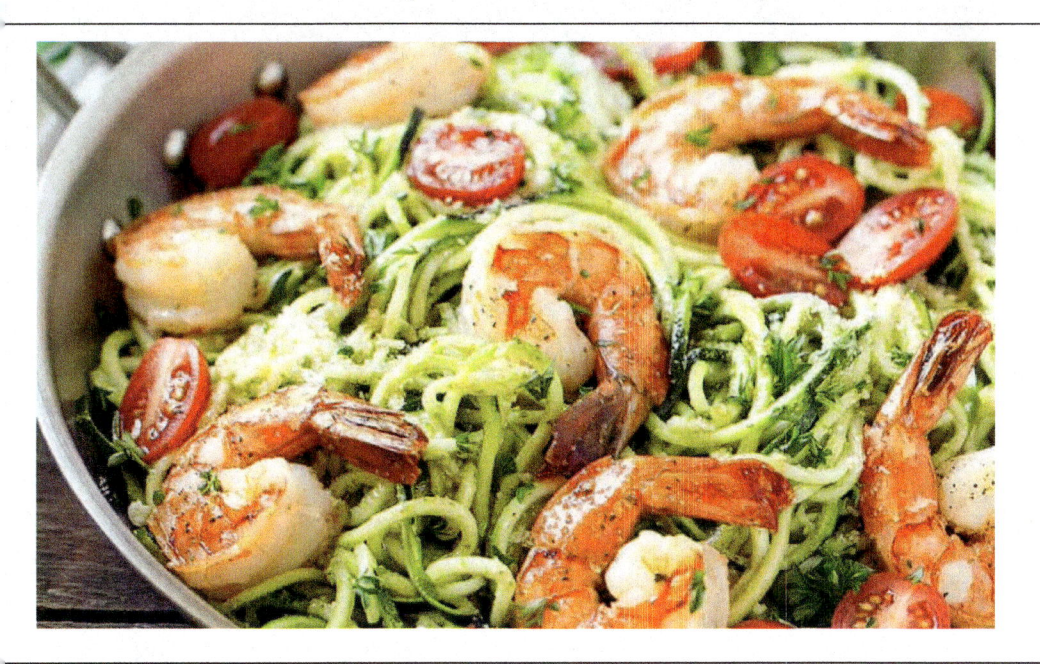

Vibe: A light and flavorful dish featuring zucchini noodles, grilled shrimp, and garlic-free pesto.

Ingredients

- Zucchini noodles (zoodles)
- Grilled shrimp
- Pesto sauce without garlic (check for FODMAP content)
- Olive oil, salt, and pepper for seasoning

Steps for Cooking:

1. In a skillet, heat olive oil over medium-high heat.
2. Add zucchini noodles and sauté until tender.
3. Season with salt and pepper.
4. Grill shrimp until cooked.
5. Toss zucchini noodles with pesto sauce (use a garlic-free variety).
6. Top with grilled shrimp.
7. Enjoy your Low FODMAP zucchini noodles with grilled shrimp and pesto.

HERB-CRUSTED LAMB CHOPS WITH MASHED PARSNIPS AND GREEN BEANS

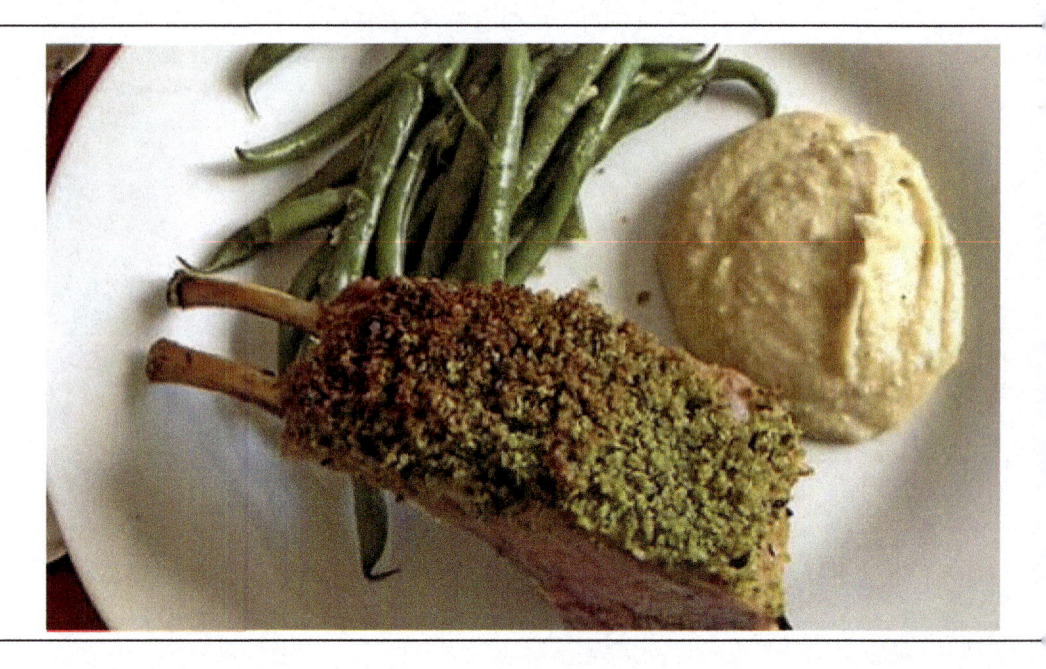

A luxurious and flavorsome dish, with herb-crusted lamb chops taking center stage, complemented by creamy mashed parsnips and crisp green beans.

Ingredients

- Lamb chops
- Fresh herbs (e.g., rosemary, thyme)
- Parsnips, peeled and boiled
- Green beans
- Olive oil, salt, and pepper for seasoning

Steps for Cooking:

1. Season lamb chops with fresh herbs, olive oil, salt, and pepper.
2. Grill or sear lamb chops until cooked to your liking.
3. Mash boiled parsnips and season with salt and pepper.
4. Steam green beans until tender.
5. Serve herb-crusted lamb chops with mashed parsnips and green beans.
6. Enjoy your Low FODMAP herb-crusted lamb chops with mashed parsnips and green beans.

DAY 16

GLUTEN-FREE WAFFLES WITH MAPLE SYRUP AND A SIDE OF LACTOSE-FREE YOGURT

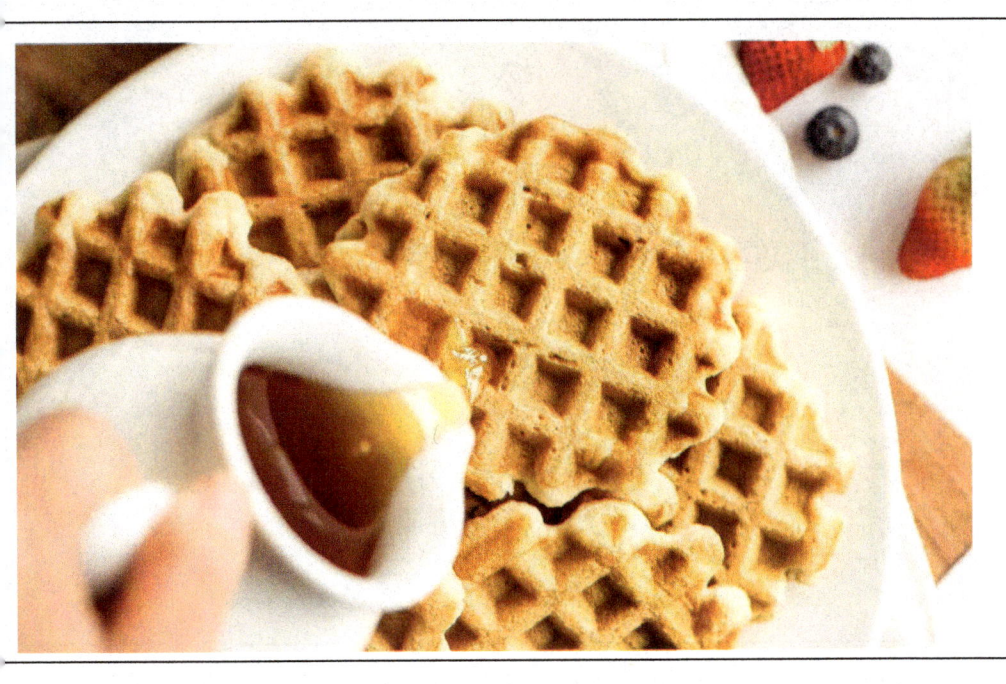

Vibe: Delicious gluten-free waffles drizzled with maple syrup and served with a side of creamy lactose-free yogurt.

Ingredients

- 2 gluten-free waffles (check label for FODMAP content)
- High-quality, very low quantity maple syrup for drizzling
- 1/2 cup lactose-free yogurt

Steps for Cooking:

1. Toast the gluten-free waffles until golden brown.
2. Drizzle maple syrup over the waffles.
3. Serve with a side of lactose-free yogurt.
4. Enjoy your Low FODMAP gluten-free waffles with maple syrup and yogurt.

BEEF AND BROCCOLI STIR-FRY WITH RICE NOODLES

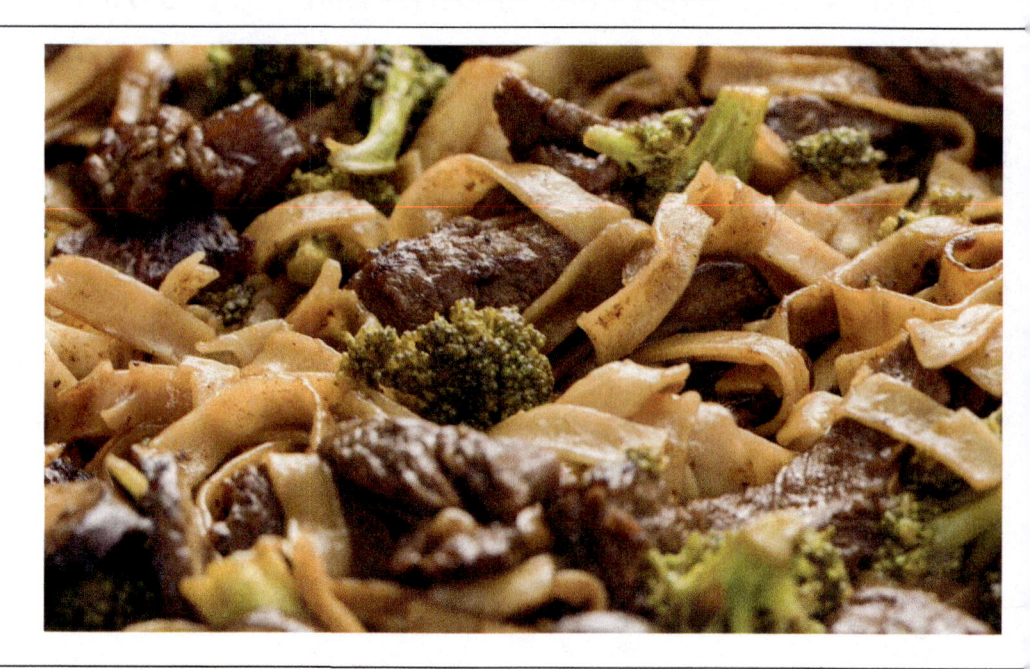

Vibe: A savory stir-fry with tender beef, broccoli, and rice noodles.

Ingredients

- Thinly sliced beef
- Broccoli florets
- Rice noodles (check for FODMAP content)
- Tamari sauce (check for FODMAP content)
- Olive oil for cooking

Steps for Cooking:

1. Cook rice noodles according to package instructions.
2. Heat a skillet or wok with olive oil over high heat.
3. Stir-fry thinly sliced beef until cooked.
4. Add broccoli florets and continue stir-frying until tender.
5. Drizzle with tamari sauce (use a Low FODMAP variety).
6. Toss with cooked rice noodles.
7. Enjoy your Low FODMAP beef and broccoli stir-fry with rice noodles.

SHRIMP AND VEGETABLE CURRY (USE A LOW FODMAP CURRY PASTE) WITH RICE

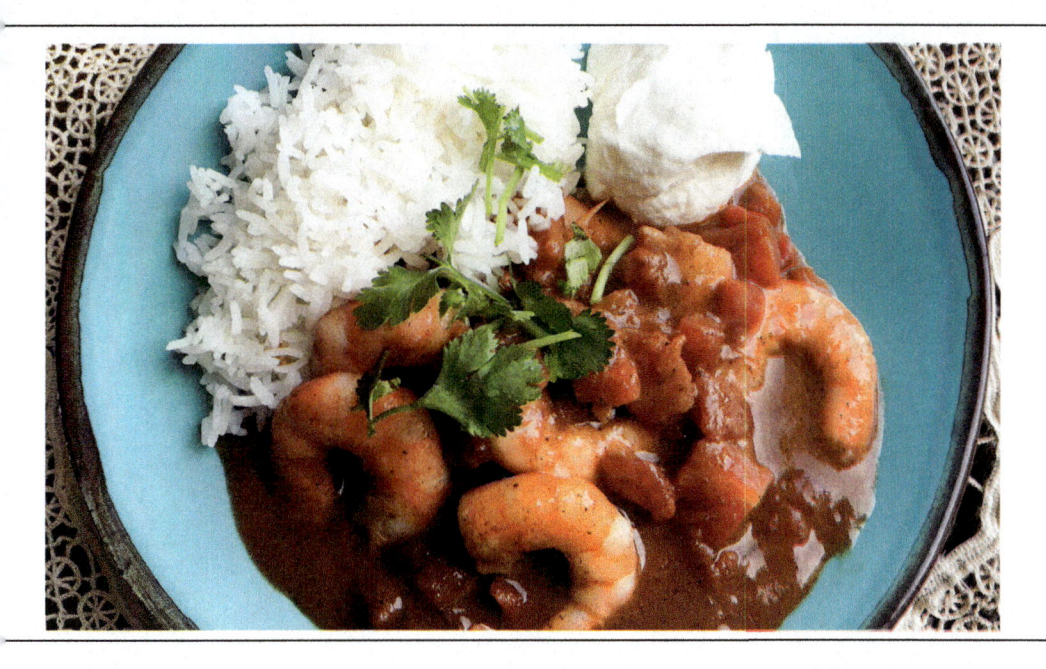

A vibrant and aromatic curry, brimming with succulent shrimp and fresh vegetables, served with fluffy rice for a comforting and exotic experience.

Ingredients

- Mixed vegetables (e.g., bell peppers, zucchini)
- Low FODMAP curry paste
- Rice (check for FODMAP content)
- Olive oil, salt, and pepper for seasoning

Steps for Cooking:

1. In a skillet, heat olive oil and sauté mixed vegetables until tender.
2. Add shrimp and cook until pink and opaque.
3. Stir in Low FODMAP curry paste and simmer until heated through.
4. Season with salt and pepper.
5. Cook rice according to package instructions (use a Low FODMAP variety).
6. Serve shrimp and vegetable curry with rice.
7. Enjoy your Low FODMAP shrimp and vegetable curry with rice.

DAY 17

OMELETTE WITH SPINACH, SWISS CHEESE, AND CHERRY TOMATOES

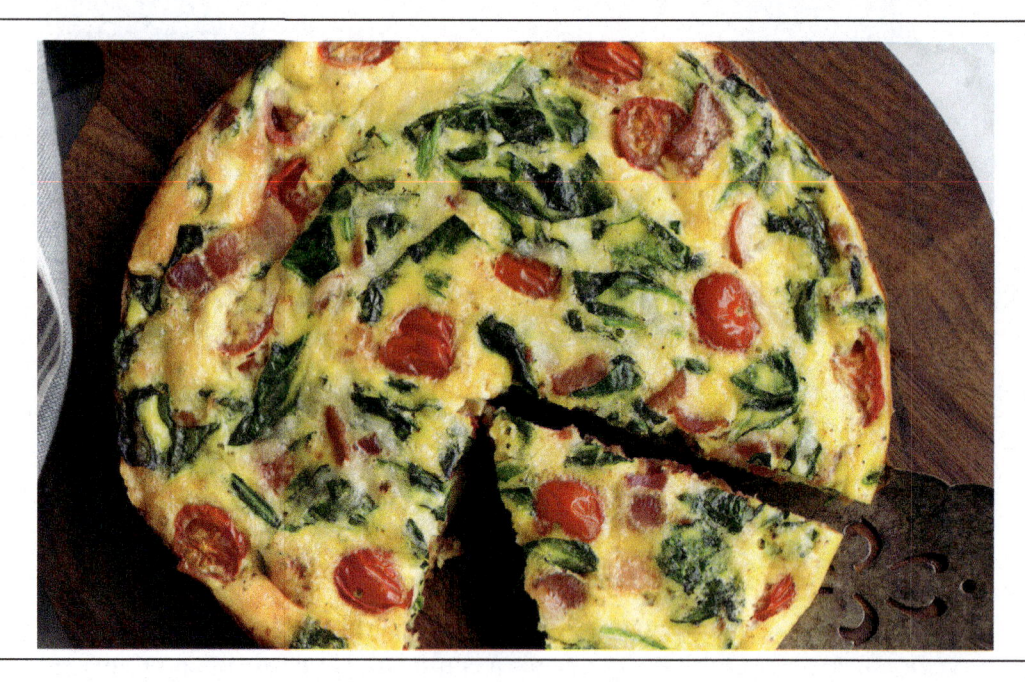

Vibe: A flavorful and satisfying omelette with the goodness of spinach, Swiss cheese, and cherry tomatoes.

Ingredients

- 2 large eggs
- 1/2 cup fresh spinach leaves
- 1/4 cup Swiss cheese, grated
- 1/4 cup cherry tomatoes, halved
- Salt and pepper to taste
- Olive oil for cooking

Steps for Cooking:

1. In a bowl, whisk the eggs until well beaten.
2. Heat a non-stick skillet over medium heat with a drizzle of olive oil.
3. Pour the beaten eggs into the skillet.
4. Sprinkle grated Swiss cheese evenly over the eggs.
5. Add cherry tomato halves.
6. Season with salt and pepper to taste.
7. Cook until the eggs are set.
8. Fold the omelette in half.
9. Serve hot and enjoy your Low FODMAP omelette with spinach, Swiss cheese, and cherry tomatoes.

GRILLED PORK CHOPS WITH MASHED POTATOES (USING LACTOSE-FREE MILK) AND SAUTÉED SPINACH

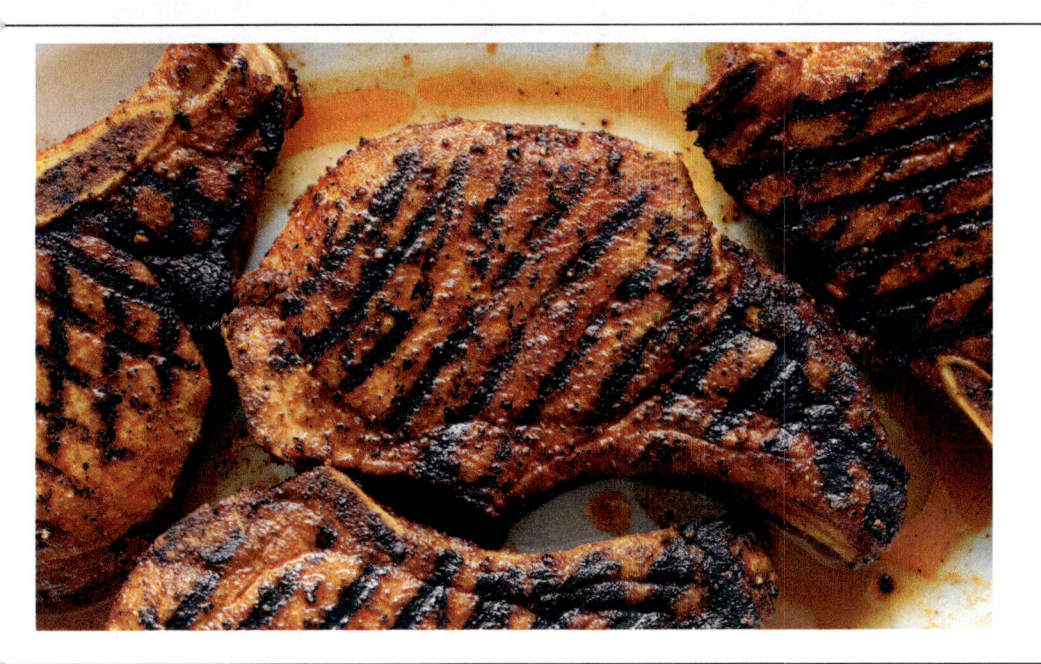

Vibe: A hearty dinner with grilled pork chops, creamy mashed potatoes made with lactose-free milk, and sautéed spinach.

Ingredients

- Grilled pork chops
- Potatoes (check for FODMAP content)
- Lactose-free milk
- Olive oil, salt, and pepper for seasoning
- Spinach leaves

Steps for Cooking:

1. Grill pork chops until cooked to your liking.
2. Peel and boil potatoes until tender.
3. Mash potatoes with lactose-free milk, olive oil, salt, and pepper until creamy.
4. Sauté spinach leaves until wilted.
5. Serve grilled pork chops with mashed potatoes and sautéed spinach.
6. Enjoy your Low FODMAP grilled pork chops with creamy mashed potatoes and spinach.

GRILLED EGGPLANT PARMESAN WITH A SIDE SALAD
(USE LOW FODMAP DRESSING)

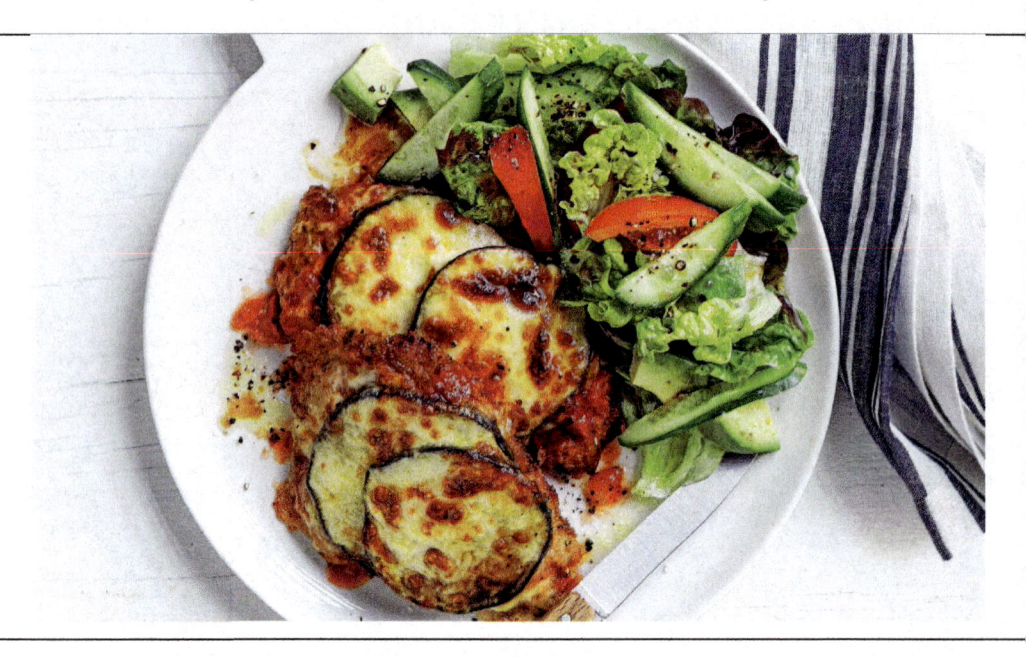

A delightful vegetarian twist on a classic, featuring grilled eggplant slices layered with cheese and sauce, accompanied by a fresh and crisp salad.

Ingredients

- Eggplant slices
- Tomato sauce (check for FODMAP content)
- Mozzarella cheese (if tolerated)
- Fresh basil leaves
- Mixed salad greens
- Low FODMAP salad dressing
- Olive oil, salt, and pepper for seasoning

Steps for Cooking:

1. Preheat the grill.
2. Grill eggplant slices until tender and lightly charred.
3. Layer grilled eggplant with tomato sauce and mozzarella cheese (if tolerated).
4. Sprinkle with fresh basil leaves.
5. In a separate bowl, toss mixed salad greens with low FODMAP salad dressing.
6. Season with olive oil, salt, and pepper.
7. Serve grilled eggplant Parmesan with a side salad.
8. Enjoy your Low FODMAP grilled eggplant Parmesan with a side salad.

DAY 18

POLENTA WITH GRILLED ZUCCHINI AND A POACHED EGG

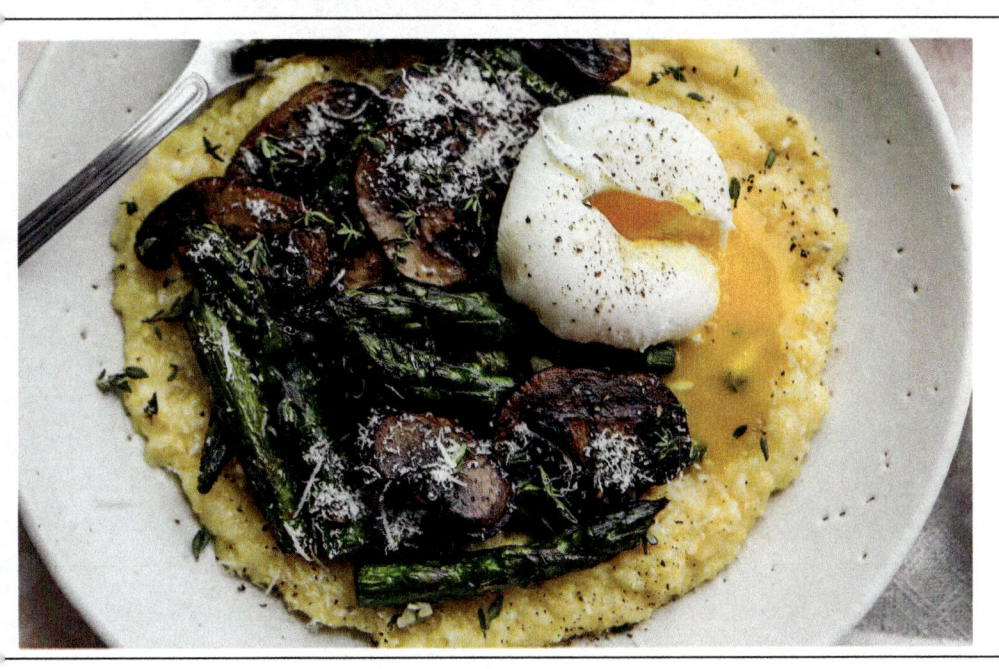

Vibe: A warm and comforting breakfast featuring polenta, grilled zucchini, and a perfectly poached egg.

Ingredients

- 1/2 cup cooked polenta (check for FODMAP content)
- 1 small zucchini, sliced and grilled
- 1 poached egg
- Salt and pepper to taste

Steps for Cooking:

1. Prepare cooked polenta according to package instructions.
2. Grill zucchini slices until tender.
3. Poach an egg to your desired level of doneness.
4. Place the cooked polenta on a plate.
5. Top with grilled zucchini slices and the poached egg.
6. Season with salt and pepper to taste.
7. Enjoy your Low FODMAP polenta with grilled zucchini and a poached egg.

SPINACH AND TOMATO FRITTATA WITH A SIDE OF MIXED GREENS

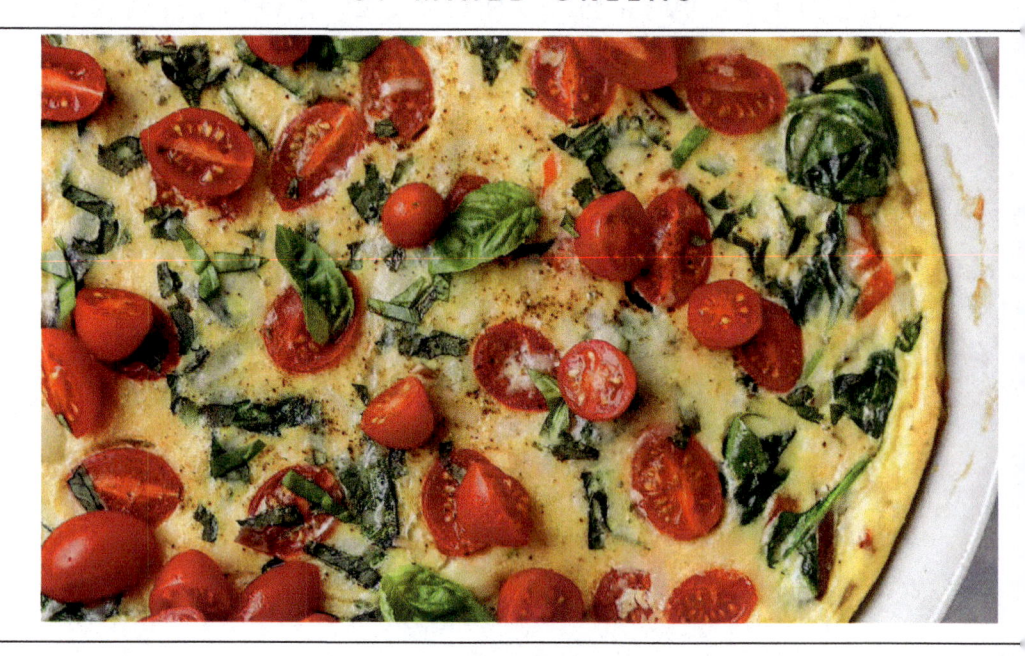

Vibe: A delicious frittata filled with spinach and tomatoes, served with a side of mixed greens.

Ingredients

- Eggs
- Fresh spinach leaves
- Tomato slices
- Olive oil, salt, and pepper for seasoning
- Mixed greens for the side

Steps for Cooking:

1. Preheat the oven to 350ºF (175ºC).
2. In an oven-safe skillet, heat olive oil over medium heat.
3. Add fresh spinach leaves and sauté until wilted.
4. Arrange tomato slices on top of the spinach.
5. In a bowl, whisk eggs and season with salt and pepper.
6. Pour the egg mixture over the spinach and tomatoes.
7. Cook on the stovetop for a few minutes until the edges set.
8. Transfer the skillet to the oven and bake for about 15 minutes or until the frittata is cooked through.
9. Serve with a side of mixed greens.
10. Enjoy your Low FODMAP spinach and tomato frittata.

TURKEY AND CHEDDAR CHEESE STUFFED BELL PEPPERS

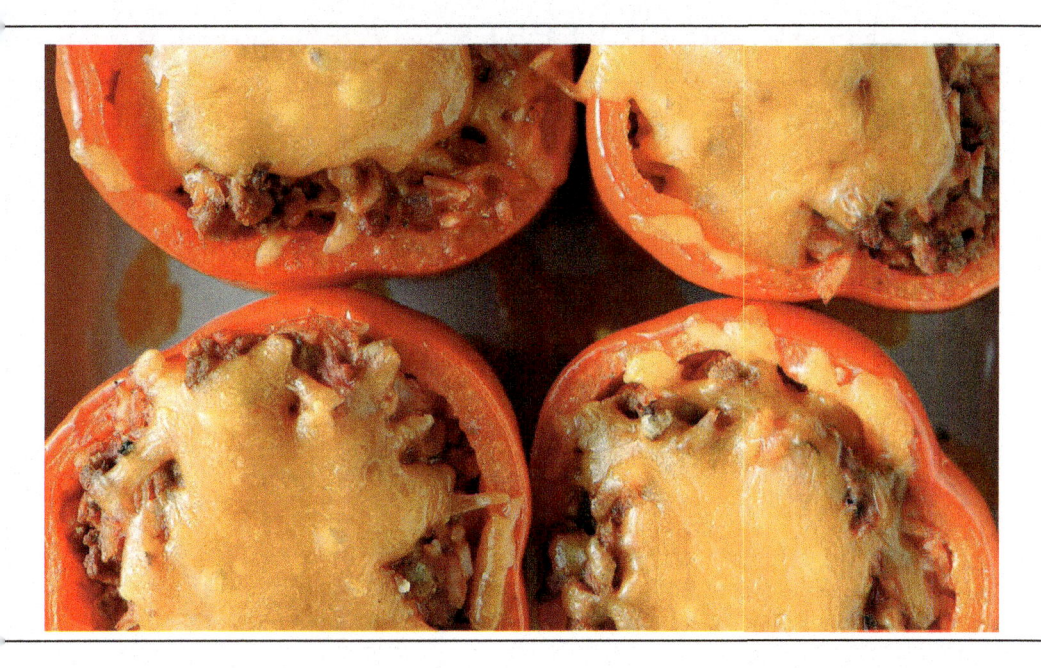

A cheesy and satisfying dish, where bell peppers are generously filled with a flavorful mixture of turkey and cheddar, creating a comforting meal.

Ingredients

- Bell peppers
- Ground turkey
- Cheddar cheese (if tolerated)
- Olive oil, salt, and pepper for seasoning

Steps for Cooking:

1. Preheat the oven to 375°F (190°C).
2. Cut the tops off the bell peppers and remove the seeds.
3. In a skillet, cook ground turkey in olive oil until browned.
4. Stir in cheddar cheese (if tolerated) until melted and combined.
5. Season with salt and pepper.
6. Stuff the bell peppers with the turkey and cheddar cheese mixture.
7. Place the stuffed bell peppers in a baking dish.
8. Bake for about 25-30 minutes or until the bell peppers are tender.
9. Enjoy your Low FODMAP turkey and cheddar cheese stuffed bell peppers.

DAY 19

BREAKFAST TACOS WITH SCRAMBLED EGGS, BELL PEPPERS, AND SALSA

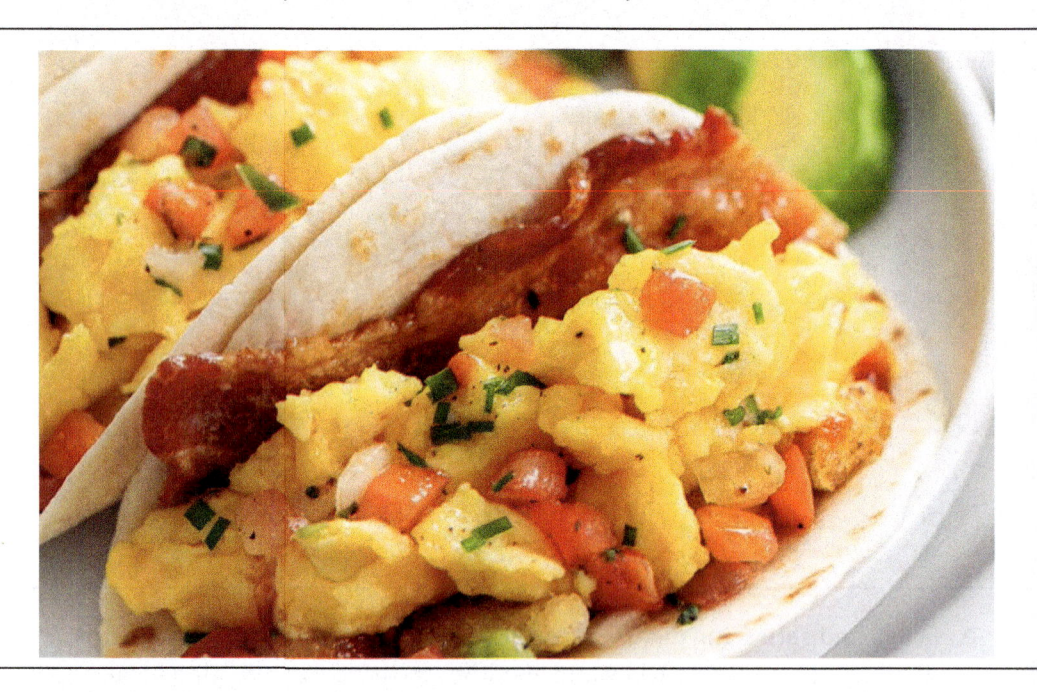

Vibe: A flavorful breakfast taco with scrambled eggs, bell peppers, and zesty salsa.

Ingredients

- 2 corn tortillas
- 4 large eggs, scrambled
- 1/4 cup diced red bell peppers
- 1/4 cup diced green bell peppers
- Salsa (check ingredients for FODMAPs)
- Salt and pepper to taste

Steps for Cooking:

1. Warm corn tortillas in a dry skillet or microwave.
2. In a separate skillet, scramble the eggs until cooked.
3. Sauté diced red and green bell peppers until slightly softened.
4. Fill each tortilla with scrambled eggs and sautéed bell peppers.
5. Top with salsa.
6. Season with salt and pepper to taste.
7. Serve and enjoy your Low FODMAP breakfast tacos.

LOW FODMAP MARGHERITA PIZZA (HOMEMADE WITH LOW FODMAP INGREDIENTS)

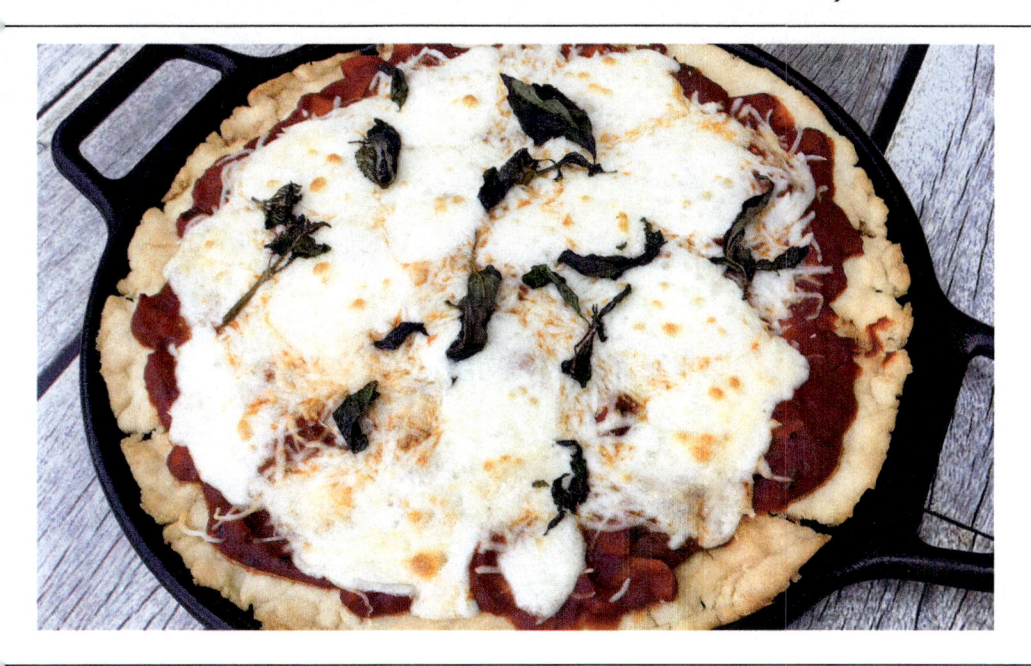

Vibe: Classic Margherita pizza made with gluten-free crust, low FODMAP tomato sauce, lactose-free mozzarella, and fresh basil.

Ingredients

- 1 gluten-free pizza crust (check for FODMAP content)
- 1/2 cup low FODMAP tomato sauce
- 1 cup lactose-free mozzarella cheese, shredded
- Fresh basil leaves for garnish
- Olive oil for drizzling (optional)
- Salt and pepper to taste

Steps for Cooking:

1. Preheat your oven to the temperature specified on the pizza crust packaging.
2. Spread low FODMAP tomato sauce evenly over the pizza crust.
3. Sprinkle lactose-free mozzarella cheese on top of the sauce.
4. Bake the pizza in the oven according to the crust's instructions or until the cheese is bubbly and golden.
5. Remove the pizza from the oven and garnish with fresh basil leaves.
6. Drizzle with a bit of olive oil if desired.
7. Season with salt and pepper to taste.
8. Slice and enjoy your homemade Low FODMAP Margherita Pizza.

ROASTED HERB TURKEY WITH BAKED ACORN SQUASH AND MIXED GREENS

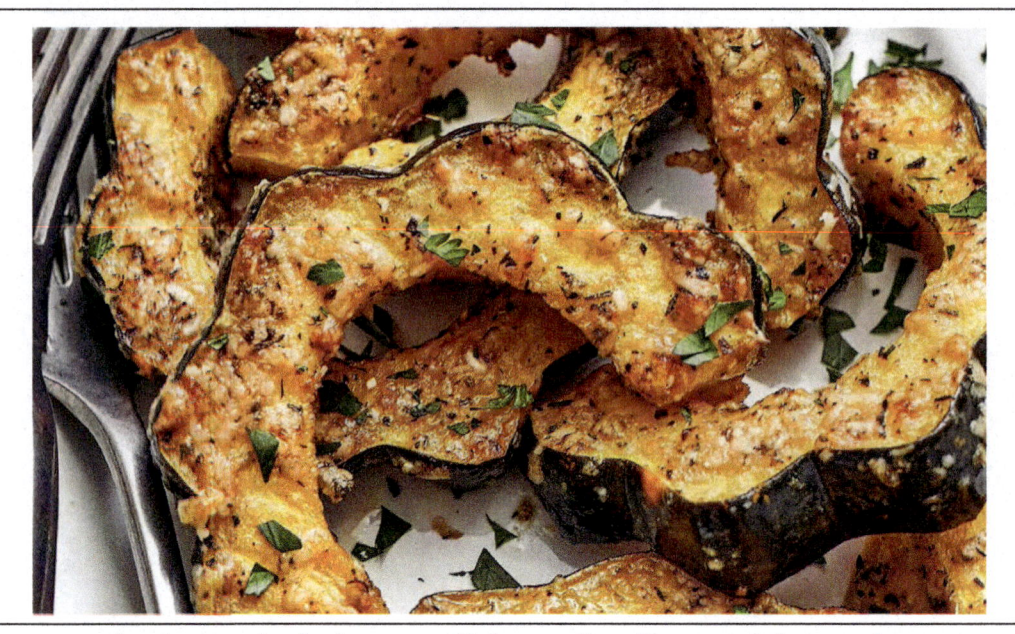

A festive and wholesome dish, perfect for special occasions, featuring herb-infused roasted turkey alongside sweet acorn squash and a bed of mixed greens.

Ingredients

- Bell peppers
- Ground turkey
- Cheddar cheese (if tolerated)
- Olive oil, salt, and pepper for seasoning

Steps for Cooking:

1. Preheat the oven to 375°F (190°C).
2. Season turkey with fresh herbs, olive oil, salt, and pepper.
3. Roast the turkey until cooked through and golden brown.
4. Cut acorn squash into wedges, season with olive oil, salt, and pepper, and bake until tender.
5. Toss mixed salad greens with olive oil, salt, and pepper.
6. Serve roasted herb turkey with baked acorn squash and mixed greens.
7. Enjoy your Low FODMAP roasted herb turkey with baked acorn squash and mixed greens.

DAY 20

LACTOSE-FREE YOGURT PARFAIT WITH KIWI AND PUMPKIN SEEDS

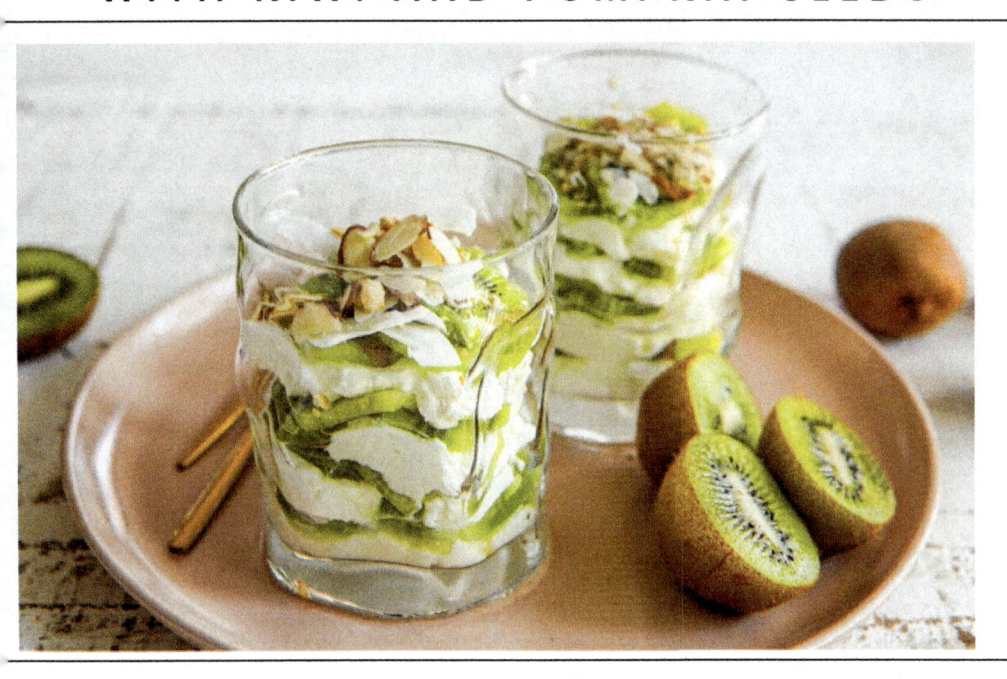

Vibe: A creamy and fruity parfait with a delightful crunch of pumpkin seeds.

Ingredients

- 1 cup lactose-free yogurt
- 1 kiwi, sliced
- 1 tablespoon pumpkin seeds

Steps for Cooking:

1. In a glass or bowl, layer half of the lactose-free yogurt.
2. Add half of the sliced kiwi on top of the yogurt.
3. Sprinkle pumpkin seeds over the kiwi.
4. Repeat the layers with the remaining ingredients.
5. Finish with a few kiwi slices and a sprinkle of pumpkin seeds on top.
6. Enjoy your Low FODMAP yogurt parfait with kiwi and pumpkin seeds.

CHICKEN CAESAR SALAD WITH HOMEMADE LOW FODMAP CAESAR DRESSING

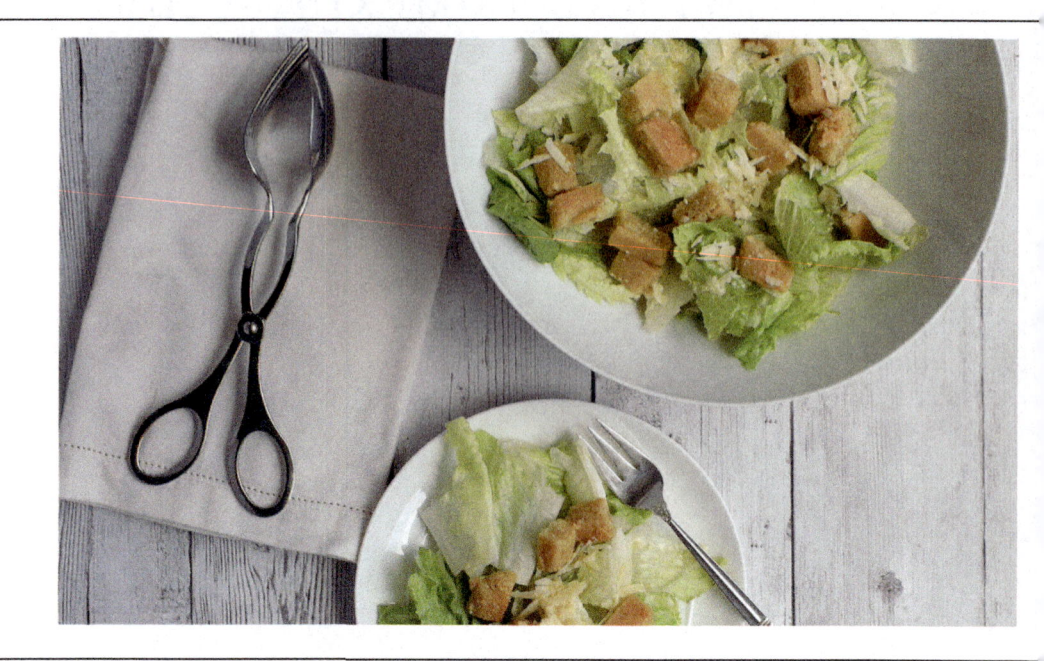

Vibe: A classic Chicken Caesar salad with a homemade low FODMAP Caesar dressing.

Ingredients

- Grilled chicken breast, sliced
- Romaine lettuce leaves
- Homemade low FODMAP Caesar dressing (e.g., made with lactose-free yogurt, Dijon mustard, lemon juice, anchovy paste)
- Croutons (check for FODMAP content)
- Grated Parmesan cheese (check for FODMAP content)

Steps for Cooking:

1. Arrange romaine lettuce leaves on a plate.
2. Top with sliced grilled chicken.
3. Drizzle with homemade low FODMAP Caesar dressing.
4. Add croutons (if tolerated) and sprinkle with grated Parmesan cheese.
5. Enjoy your Low FODMAP Chicken Caesar salad.

BAKED PORK LOIN WITH MASHED POTATOES (USING LACTOSE-FREE MILK) AND GREEN BEANS

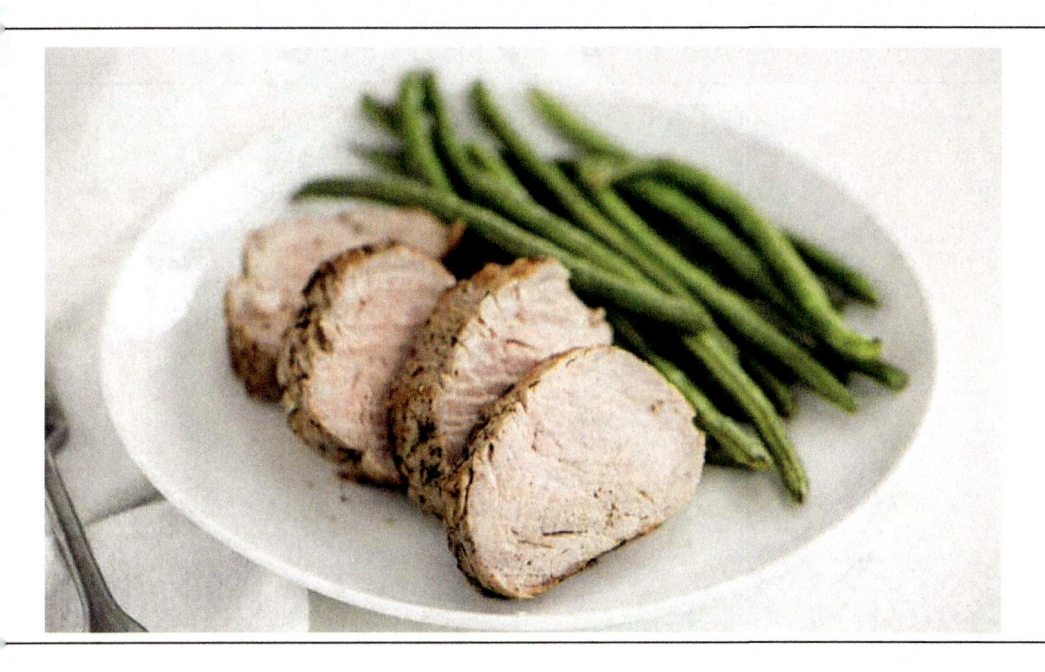

A classic and elegant dish, combining the richness of baked pork loin with the smoothness of mashed potatoes and the tenderness of asparagus.

Ingredients

- Pork loin
- Potatoes (check for FODMAP content)
- Lactose-free milk
- Asparagus
- Olive oil, salt, and pepper for seasoning

Steps for Cooking:

1. Preheat the oven to 375ºF (190ºC).
2. Season pork loin with olive oil, salt, and pepper.
3. Bake pork loin until cooked through.
4. Boil and mash potatoes, using lactose-free milk for creaminess.
5. Steam asparagus until tender.
6. Season with olive oil, salt, and pepper.
7. Serve baked pork loin with mashed potatoes and asparagus.
8. Enjoy your Low FODMAP baked pork loin with mashed potatoes and asparagus.

DAY 21

SAUTÉED KALE WITH CRISPY BACON AND A FRIED EGG

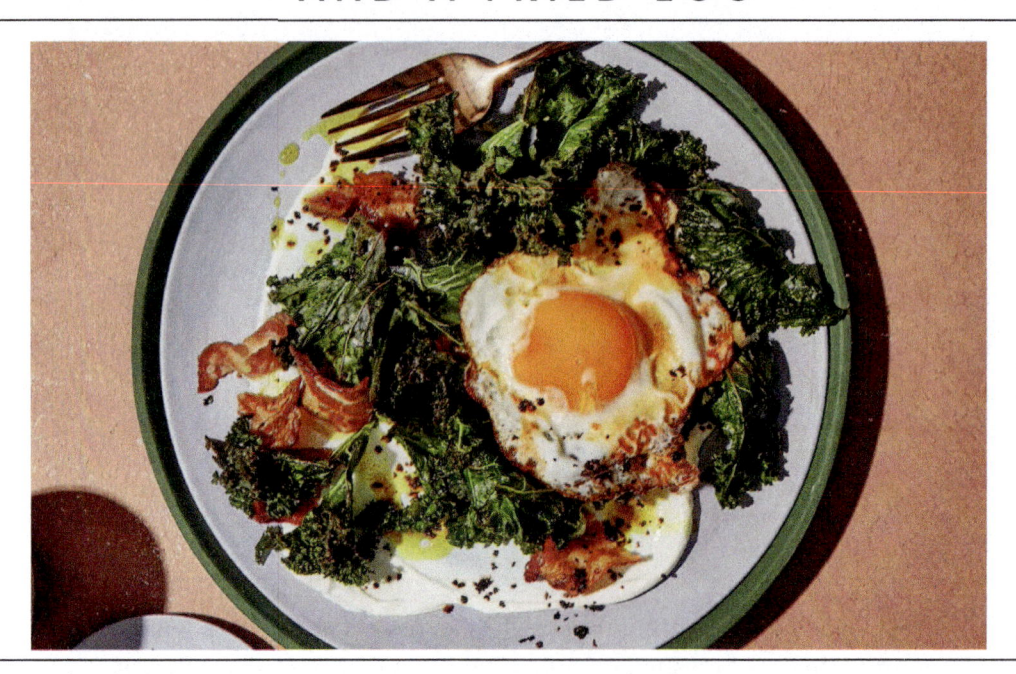

Vibe: A hearty and nutritious breakfast featuring sautéed kale, crispy bacon, and a sunny-side-up fried egg.

Ingredients

- 2 cups fresh kale leaves, destemmed and chopped
- 2 strips of bacon (check for any high FODMAP ingredients)
- 1 large egg
- Salt and pepper to taste
- Olive oil for cooking

Steps for Cooking:

1. In a skillet, cook bacon until crispy, then crumble it. Set aside.
2. In the same skillet, add a drizzle of olive oil and sauté chopped kale until wilted.
3. Season kale with salt and pepper to taste.
4. In another pan, fry an egg sunny-side up.
5. Serve sautéed kale on a plate, topped with crumbled bacon and a fried egg.
6. Enjoy your Low FODMAP sautéed kale with crispy bacon and a fried egg.

TURKEY AND CRANBERRY SANDWICH ON GLUTEN-FREE BREAD (CHECK INGREDIENTS FOR FODMAPS)

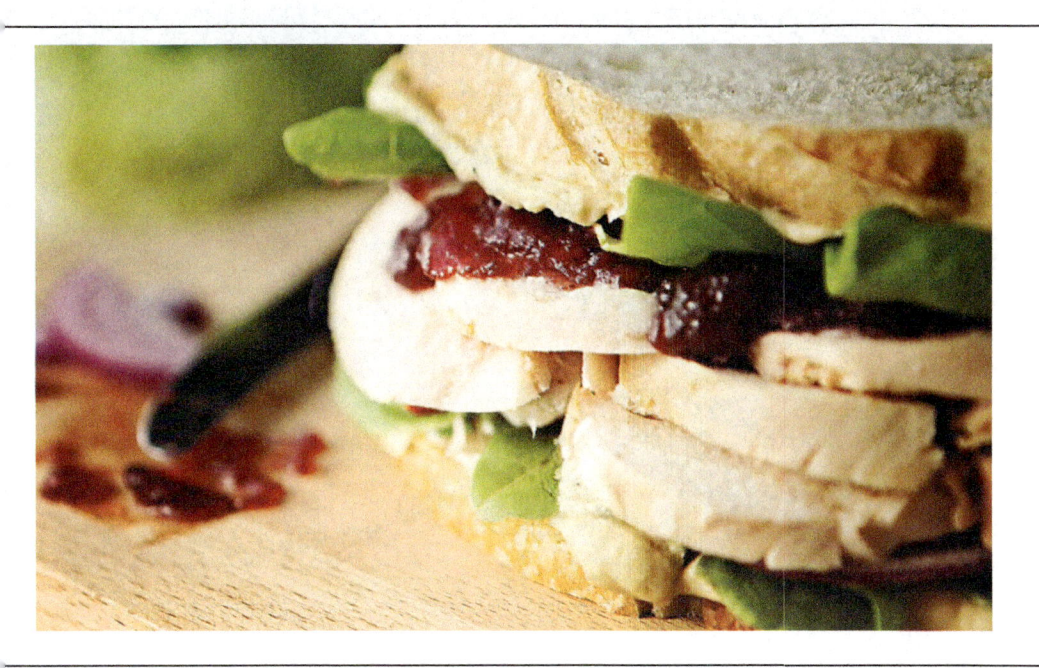

Vibe: A satisfying turkey and cranberry sandwich on gluten-free bread (ensure FODMAP-friendly ingredients).

Ingredients

- Slices of turkey
- Cranberry sauce (check for FODMAP content)
- Gluten-free bread (check for FODMAP content)
- Lettuce leaves

Steps for Cooking:

1. Assemble turkey and cranberry sauce (using a Low FODMAP variety) between slices of gluten-free bread.
2. Add lettuce leaves for freshness.
3. Slice and enjoy your Low FODMAP turkey and cranberry sandwich.

LEMON AND DILL GRILLED TROUT WITH QUINOA AND ROASTED BRUSSELS SPROUTS

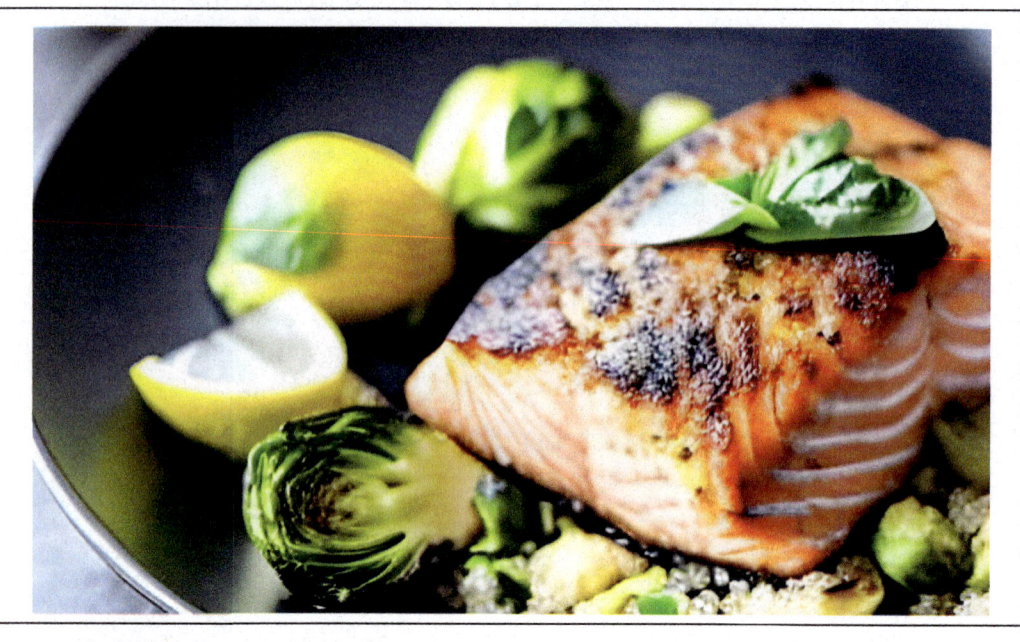

A light and refreshing meal, where the zesty flavors of lemon and dill complement the delicate trout, served with nutritious quinoa and roasted Brussels sprouts.

Ingredients

- Trout fillets
- Lemon juice
- Fresh dill
- Quinoa (check for FODMAP content)
- Brussels sprouts
- Olive oil, salt, and pepper for seasoning

Steps for Cooking:

1. Preheat the grill.
2. Season trout fillets with lemon juice and fresh dill.
3. Grill trout until flaky and cooked through.
4. Prepare quinoa according to package instructions (use a Low FODMAP variety).
5. Roast Brussels sprouts with olive oil, salt, and pepper until tender and slightly crispy.
6. Serve lemon and dill grilled trout with quinoa and roasted Brussels sprouts.
7. Enjoy your Low FODMAP lemon and dill grilled trout with quinoa and Brussels sprouts.

After completing Week 3, it's important to reflect on how your body has responded to the dietary changes. Use the following scale to rate your experiences in various aspects of your health and well-being. Rate each category from 1 to 10 (where 1 is 'no improvement' and 10 is 'significant improvement').

1. Digestive Comfort
- Question: How would you rate the overall comfort of your digestive system this week?
- Rating (1-10): _ _ _ _ _

2. Energy Levels
- Question: How do you feel about your energy levels after following the meal plan for a week?
- Rating (1-10): _ _ _ _ _

3. Sleep Quality
- Question: Have you noticed any changes in the quality of your sleep?
- Rating (1-10): _ _ _ _ _

4. Mood and Mental Clarity
- Question: How has your mood and mental clarity been affected by the dietary changes?
- Rating (1-10): _ _ _ _ _

5. Physical Comfort and Pain Levels
- Question: If you previously experienced any physical discomfort or pain, have you noticed any changes in its intensity or frequency?
- Rating (1-10): _ _ _ _ _

6. Skin Health
- Question: Have there been any noticeable changes in your skin health/appearance?
- Rating (1-10): _ _ _ _ _

7. Cravings and Appetite Control
- Question: How would you rate your control over cravings and appetite this week?
- Rating (1-10): _ _ _ _ _

8. Overall Well-being
- Question: Considering all factors, how would you rate your overall well-being after Week 1?
- Rating (1-10): _ _ _ _ _

FOR SPECIAL
notes

WEEK 4: REFLECTION AND PERSONALIZATION - CRAFTING YOUR PATH FORWARD

"Congratulations on reaching Week 4, 'Reflection and Personalization'. This final week is about reflecting on the journey you've undertaken, understanding the progress you've made, and starting to personalize your diet for the long term. You've gained valuable insights into your body's needs and are now equipped to make informed choices about your diet. This week is a celebration of your commitment and the positive steps you've taken towards lasting digestive health."

DAY 22

SMOOTHIE WITH LACTOSE-FREE KEFIR, UNRIPE BANANA, AND STRAWBERRIES

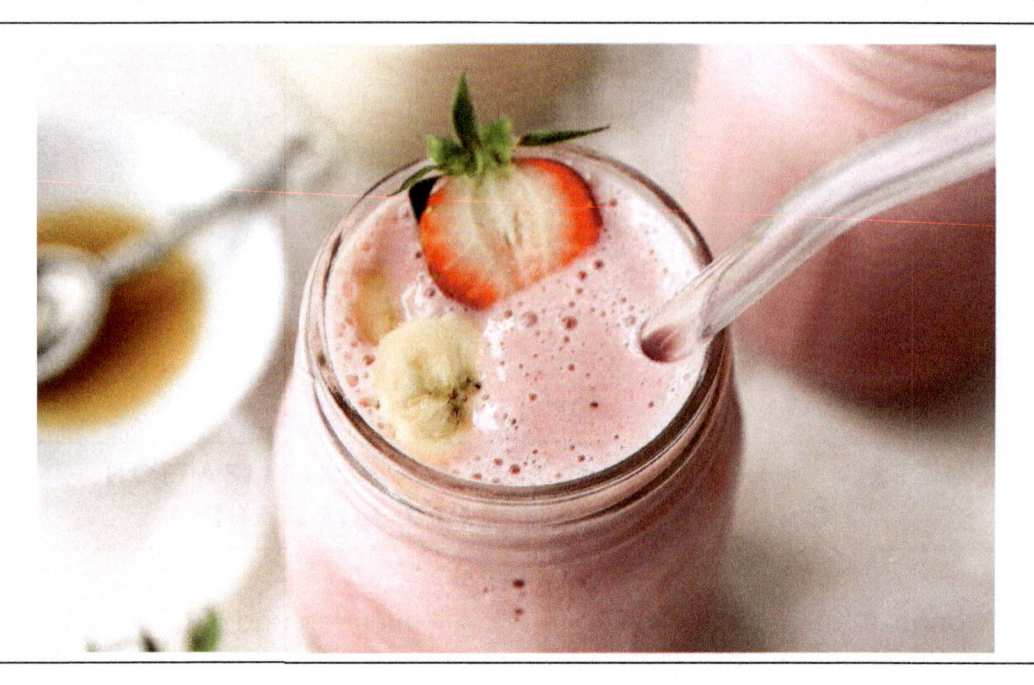

Vibe: A creamy and fruity smoothie that's gentle on the stomach.

Ingredients

- 1 cup lactose-free kefir
- 1 unripe banana
- 1/2 cup strawberries
- Ice cubes (optional)
- A drizzle of honey or maple syrup (optional for added sweetness)

Steps for Cooking:

1. Peel and slice the unripe banana.
2. In a blender, combine lactose-free kefir, sliced banana, and strawberries.
3. Add ice cubes if you prefer a colder smoothie.
4. Blend until smooth and creamy.
5. Taste and add a drizzle of honey or maple syrup if desired for extra sweetness.
6. Pour into a glass and enjoy your Low FODMAP smoothie.

GRILLED EGGPLANT AND TOMATO STACK WITH A SIDE OF ARUGULA

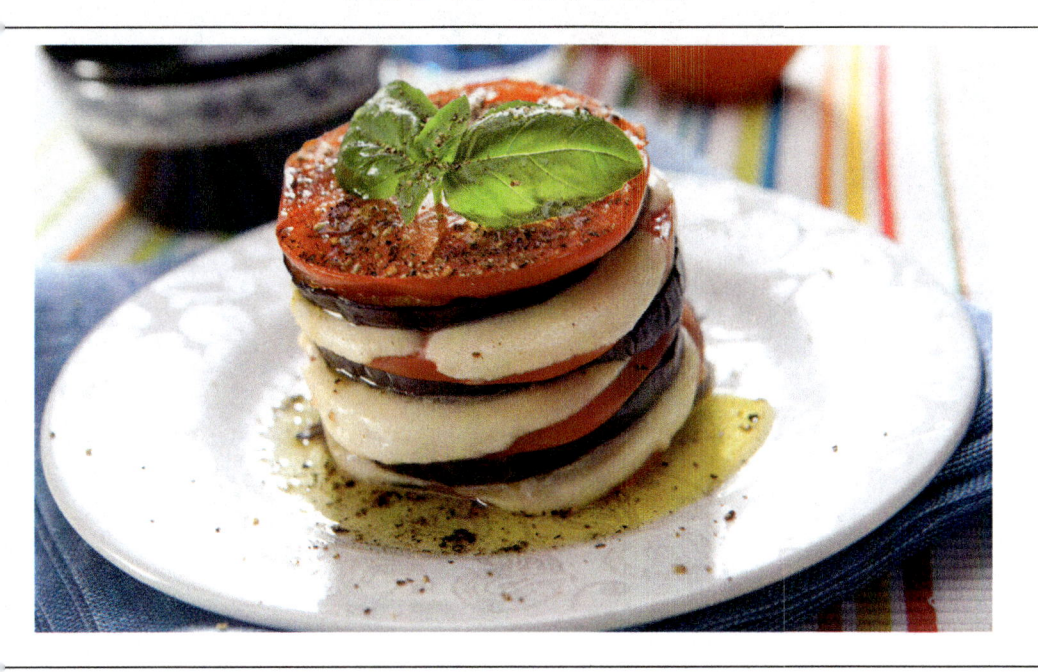

Vibe: A colorful stack of grilled eggplant and tomatoes served with a side of arugula.

Ingredients

- Slices of grilled eggplant
- Slices of grilled tomatoes
- Arugula leaves
- Olive oil, balsamic vinegar, salt, and pepper for dressing

Steps for Cooking:

1. Create stacks by layering slices of grilled eggplant and tomatoes.
2. Season with olive oil, balsamic vinegar, salt, and pepper.
3. Serve with a side of fresh arugula.
4. Enjoy your Low FODMAP grilled eggplant and tomato stack.

SPAGHETTI SQUASH WITH SAUTÉED SHRIMP AND A LEMON-BUTTER SAUCE (WITHOUT GARLIC)

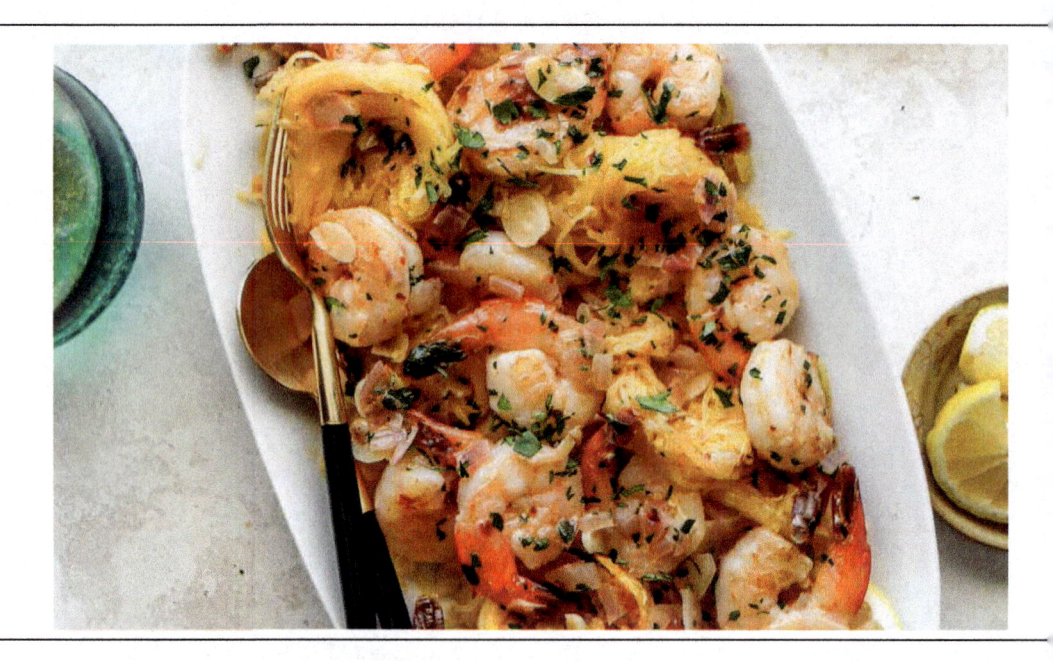

A creative and light alternative to traditional pasta, featuring spaghetti squash with succulent sautéed shrimp in a zesty lemon-butter sauce.

Ingredients

- Spaghetti squash
- Shrimp
- Butter (or dairy-free butter)
- Lemon juice and zest
- Fresh parsley
- Olive oil, salt, and pepper for seasoning

Steps for Cooking:

1. Preheat the oven to 375°F (190°C).
2. Cut the spaghetti squash in half lengthwise and remove the seeds.
3. Drizzle with olive oil, salt, and pepper, then roast until tender.
4. While the squash roasts, sauté shrimp in a pan with olive oil until pink and opaque.
5. In a separate pan, melt butter, add lemon juice and zest, and season with salt and pepper.
6. Combine cooked spaghetti squash with the lemon-butter sauce.
7. Top with sautéed shrimp and fresh parsley.
8. Enjoy your Low FODMAP spaghetti squash with sautéed shrimp and lemon-butter sauce.

DAY 23

QUINOA AND RASPBERRY MUFFINS (HOMEMADE WITH LOW FODMAP INGREDIENTS)

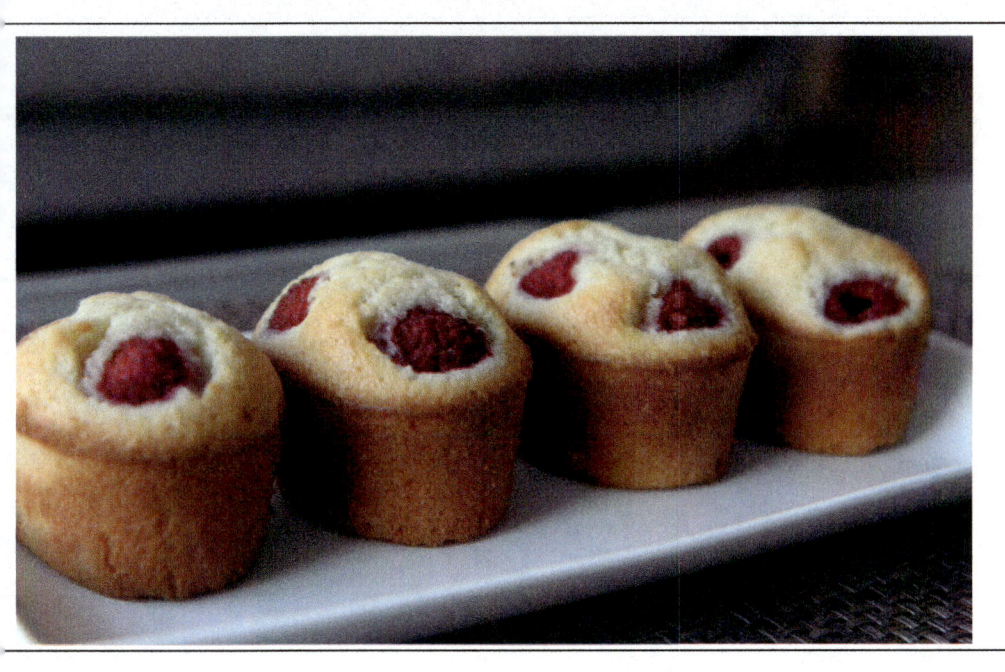

Vibe: Delicious homemade muffins featuring quinoa and raspberries.

Ingredients

- 1 cup cooked quinoa (cooled)
- 1/2 cup fresh raspberries
- 1 cup gluten-free flour (check for FODMAP content)
- 1/2 cup sugar (or a Low FODMAP sweetener)
- 2 teaspoons baking powder (check for FODMAP content)
- 1/2 teaspoon salt
- 1/2 cup lactose-free milk
- 2 large eggs
- 1/4 cup vegetable oil
- 1 teaspoon vanilla extract

Steps for Cooking:

1. Preheat the oven to 350°F (175°C). Line a muffin tin with paper liners.
2. In a mixing bowl, combine cooked quinoa and fresh raspberries.
3. In a separate bowl, whisk together gluten-free flour, sugar (or Low FODMAP sweetener), baking powder, and salt.
4. In another bowl, whisk together lactose-free milk, eggs, vegetable oil, and vanilla extract.
5. Combine the wet ingredients with the dry ingredients, then gently fold in the quinoa and raspberry mixture.
6. Fill each muffin cup about 2/3 full with the batter.
7. Bake for 18-20 minutes or until a toothpick inserted into a muffin comes out clean.
8. Allow the muffins to cool before serving.
9. Enjoy your homemade Low FODMAP quinoa and raspberry muffins.

BAKED CHICKEN THIGHS WITH ROASTED POTATOES AND GREEN BEANS

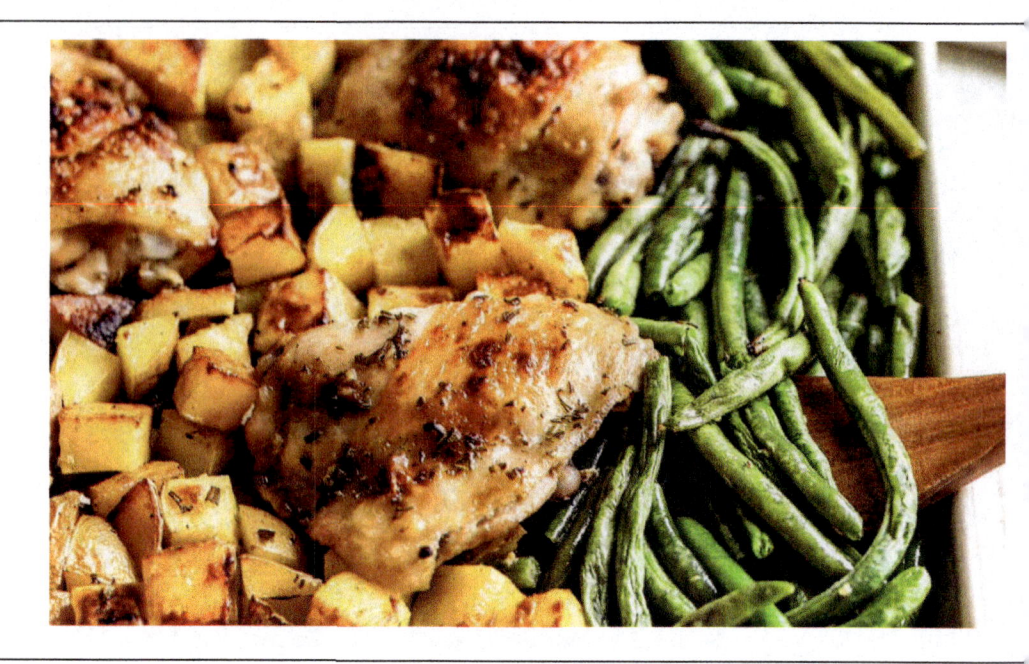

Vibe: A hearty dinner featuring baked chicken thighs, roasted potatoes, and green beans.

Ingredients

- Chicken thighs
- Potatoes (check for FODMAP content)
- Green beans
- Olive oil, salt, and pepper for seasoning

Steps for Cooking:

1. Preheat the oven to 375°F (190°C).
2. Season chicken thighs with olive oil, salt, and pepper.
3. Arrange chicken thighs, potatoes, and green beans on a baking sheet.
4. Bake for about 30-35 minutes or until the chicken is cooked through, and the potatoes and green beans are tender.
5. Serve and enjoy your Low FODMAP baked chicken thighs with roasted potatoes and green beans.

TERIYAKI CHICKEN WITH A SIDE OF GRILLED ZUCCHINI AND RICE

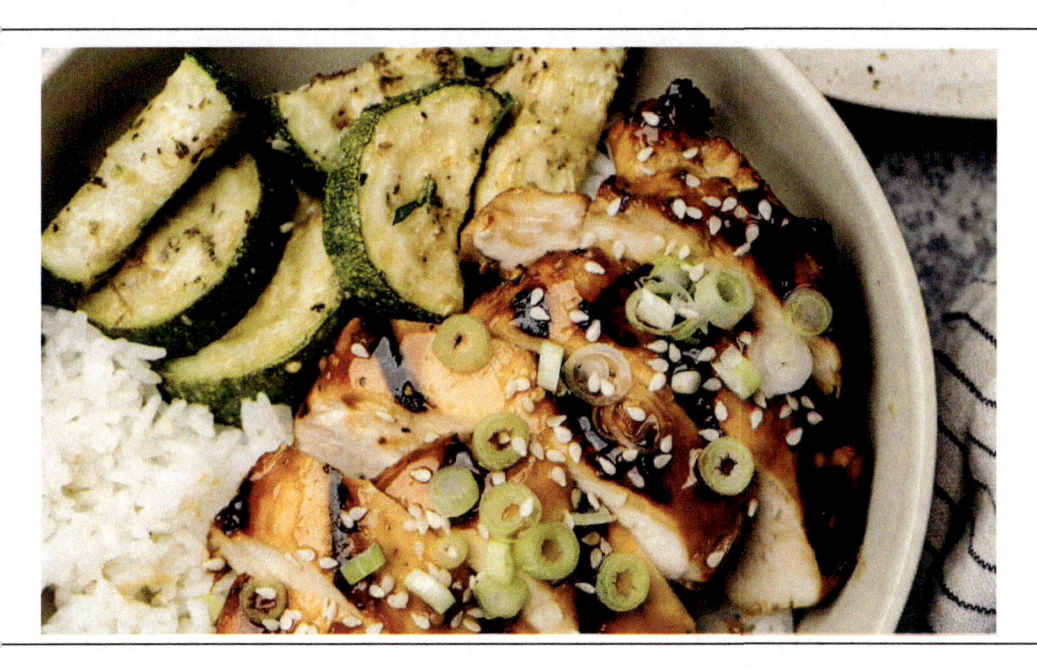

A sweet and savory delight, combining the classic taste of teriyaki chicken with the charred goodness of grilled zucchini, served alongside fluffy rice.

Ingredients

- Chicken pieces (e.g., chicken breast, chicken thighs)
- Teriyaki sauce (check for FODMAP content)
- Zucchini slices
- Rice (check for FODMAP content)
- Olive oil, salt, and pepper for seasoning

Steps for Cooking:

1. Marinate chicken pieces in teriyaki sauce.
2. Grill or cook the chicken until fully cooked.
3. Grill zucchini slices until tender and grill marks appear.
4. Cook rice according to package instructions (use a Low FODMAP variety).
5. Serve teriyaki chicken with grilled zucchini and rice.
6. Enjoy your Low FODMAP teriyaki chicken with grilled zucchini and rice.

DAY 24

BAKED EGGS WITH TOMATOES, BASIL, AND PARMESAN CHEESE

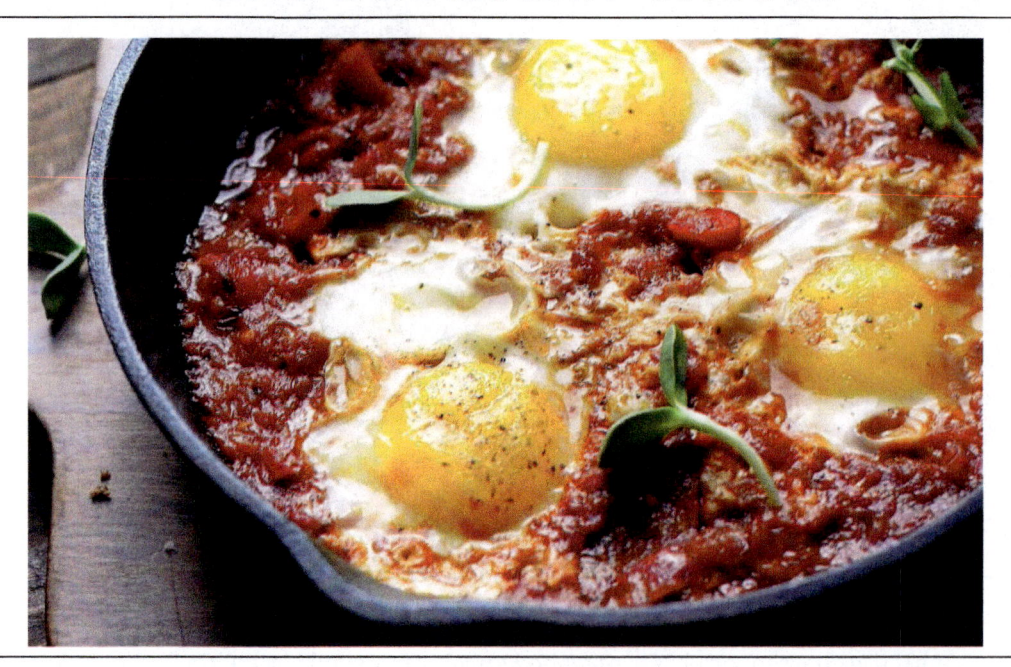

Vibe: A delightful and savory baked egg dish with the flavors of tomatoes, basil, and Parmesan cheese.

Ingredients

- 2 large eggs
- 1/2 cup diced tomatoes (remove seeds)
- Fresh basil leaves, chopped
- Grated Parmesan cheese (check for FODMAP content)
- Salt and pepper to taste
- Olive oil for greasing

Steps for Cooking:

1. Preheat the oven to 375°F (190°C). Grease a small baking dish with olive oil.
2. Crack two eggs into the greased baking dish.
3. Scatter diced tomatoes and chopped fresh basil around the eggs.
4. Sprinkle grated Parmesan cheese over the eggs and toppings.
5. Season with salt and pepper to taste.
6. Bake for about 12-15 minutes or until the egg whites are set but the yolks are still slightly runny (adjust baking time for desired yolk consistency).
7. Remove from the oven and let it cool slightly.

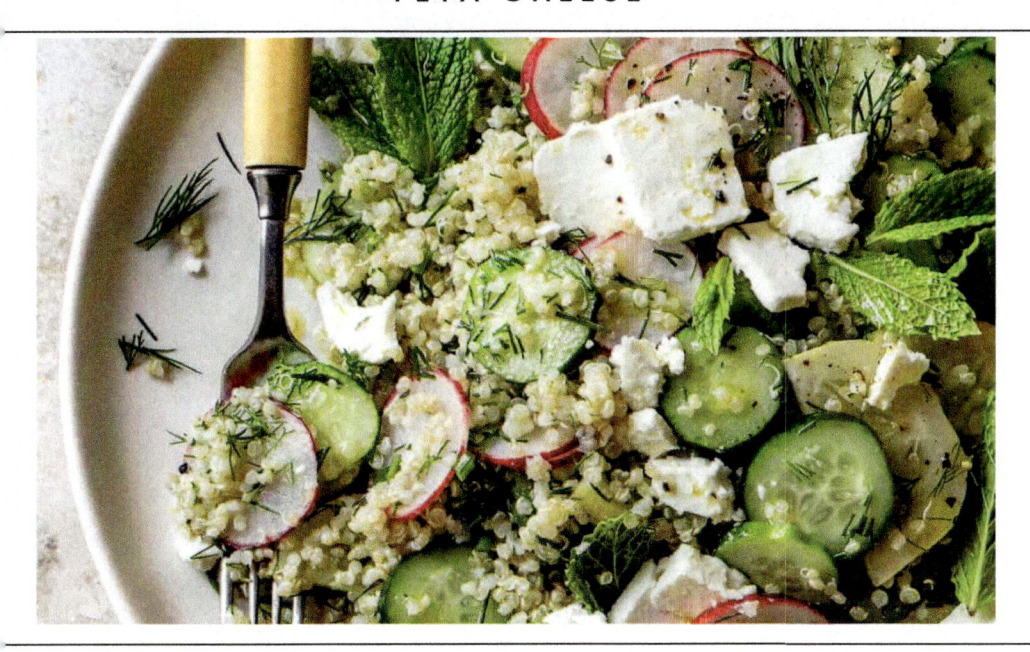

QUINOA AND CUCUMBER SALAD WITH DILL AND FETA CHEESE

Vibe: A refreshing quinoa and cucumber salad with dill and feta cheese.

Ingredients

- Cooked quinoa (check for FODMAP content)
- Sliced cucumbers
- Fresh dill leaves
- Crumbled feta cheese (check for FODMAP content)
- Olive oil, lemon juice, salt, and pepper for dressing
- Radish

Steps for Cooking:

1. In a bowl, combine cooked quinoa, sliced cucumbers, fresh dill leaves, and crumbled feta cheese.
2. Drizzle with olive oil and lemon juice.
3. Season with salt and pepper to taste.
4. Toss to combine.
5. Enjoy your Low FODMAP quinoa and cucumber salad with dill and feta cheese.

PAN-SEARED DUCK BREAST WITH SAUTÉED SWISS CHARD AND MASHED CARROTS

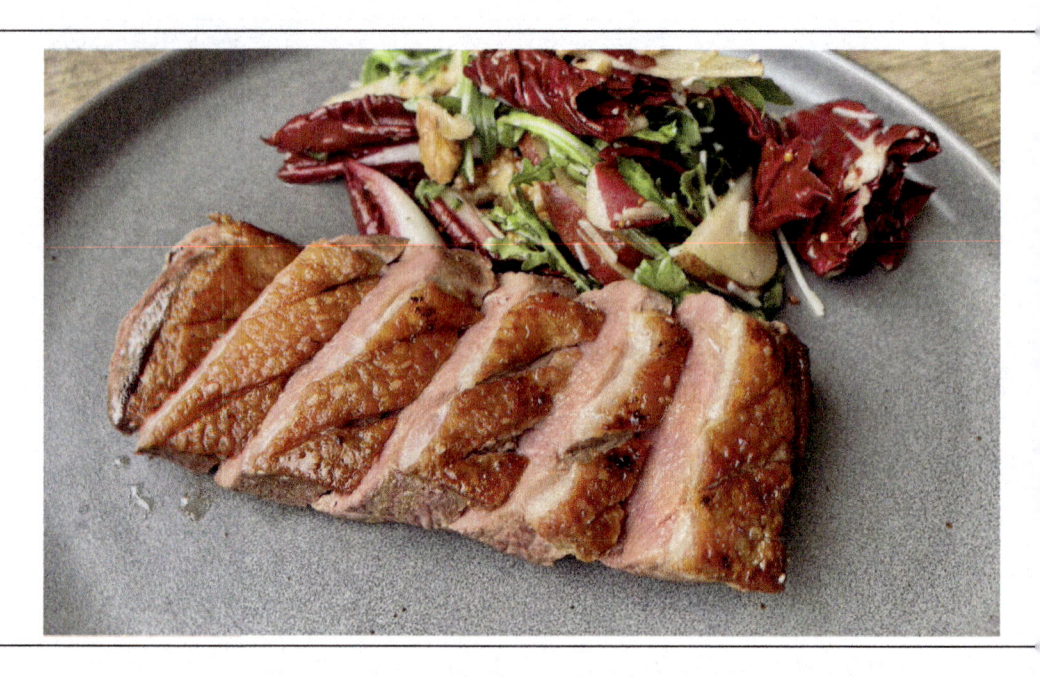

An upscale and sophisticated meal, featuring rich and flavorful duck breast, paired with nutritious Swiss chard and smoothly mashed carrots.

Ingredients

- Duck breast
- Swiss chard leaves
- Carrots
- Dairy-free milk (e.g., almond milk)
- Olive oil, salt, and pepper for seasoning

Steps for Cooking:

1. Score the duck breast skin and season with salt and pepper.
2. Sear the duck breast, skin side down, in a hot skillet until crispy.
3. Flip and cook until desired doneness is achieved.
4. Sauté Swiss chard in olive oil until wilted.
5. Boil and mash carrots, adding dairy-free milk for creaminess.
6. Season with salt and pepper.
7. Serve pan-seared duck breast with sautéed Swiss chard and mashed carrots.
8. Enjoy your Low FODMAP pan-seared duck breast with Swiss chard and mashed carrots.

DAY 25

RICE PUDDING MADE WITH LACTOSE-FREE MILK AND A SPRINKLE OF CINNAMON

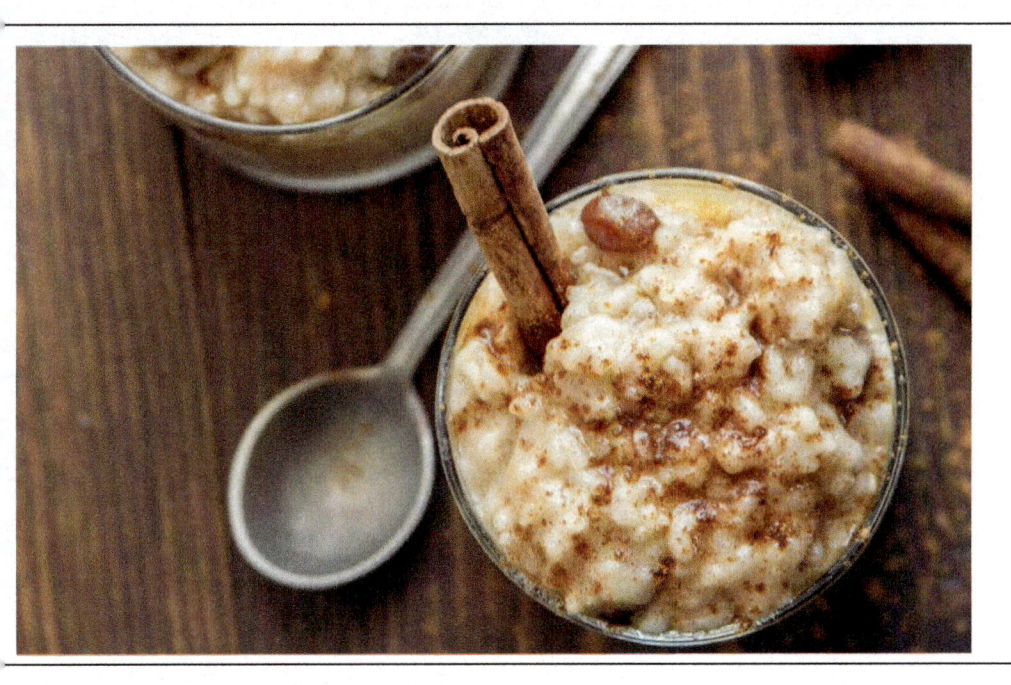

Vibe: A comforting and creamy rice pudding with a hint of cinnamon.

Ingredients

- 1 cup cooked rice (check for FODMAP content)
- 1 1/2 cups lactose-free milk
- 2 tablespoons sugar (or a Low FODMAP sweetener)
- 1/2 teaspoon ground cinnamon
- A pinch of salt
- 1/2 teaspoon vanilla extract

Steps for Cooking:

1. In a saucepan, combine cooked rice, lactose-free milk, sugar (or Low FODMAP sweetener), ground cinnamon, and a pinch of salt.
2. Heat the mixture over medium-low heat, stirring constantly.
3. Simmer for about 20-25 minutes, or until the rice absorbs the milk and the mixture thickens.
4. Remove from heat and stir in vanilla extract.
5. Let it cool slightly, and sprinkle with additional cinnamon before serving.
6. Enjoy your homemade Low FODMAP rice pudding with cinnamon.

BAKED HAM AND SWISS CHEESE ROLL-UPS WITH A SIDE OF SLICED CUCUMBERS

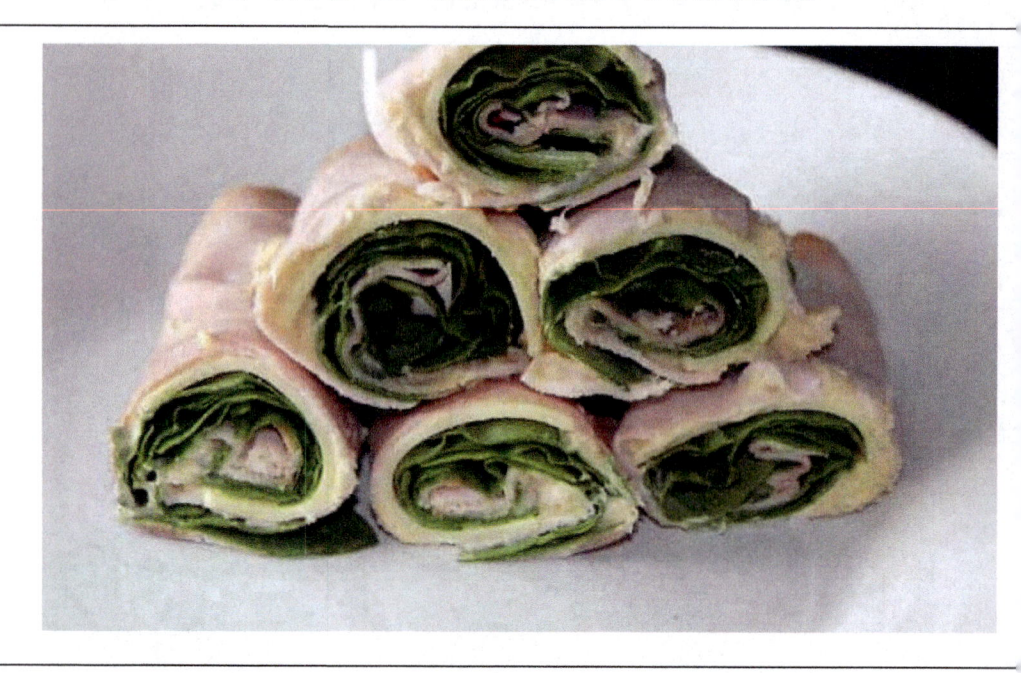

Vibe: Savory baked ham and Swiss cheese roll-ups, paired with crisp sliced cucumbers.

Ingredients

- Slices of ham
- Swiss cheese slices (check for FODMAP content)
- Sliced cucumbers
- Toothpicks (for securing roll-ups)
- spinach

Steps for Cooking:

1. Lay out slices of ham.
2. Place a slice of Swiss cheese on each slice of ham.
3. Roll up the ham and cheese slices and secure with toothpicks.
4. Serve with crisp sliced cucumbers on the side.
5. Enjoy your Low FODMAP baked ham and Swiss cheese roll-ups.

LOW FODMAP CHICKEN ALFREDO (HOMEMADE WITH LOW FODMAP INGREDIENTS)

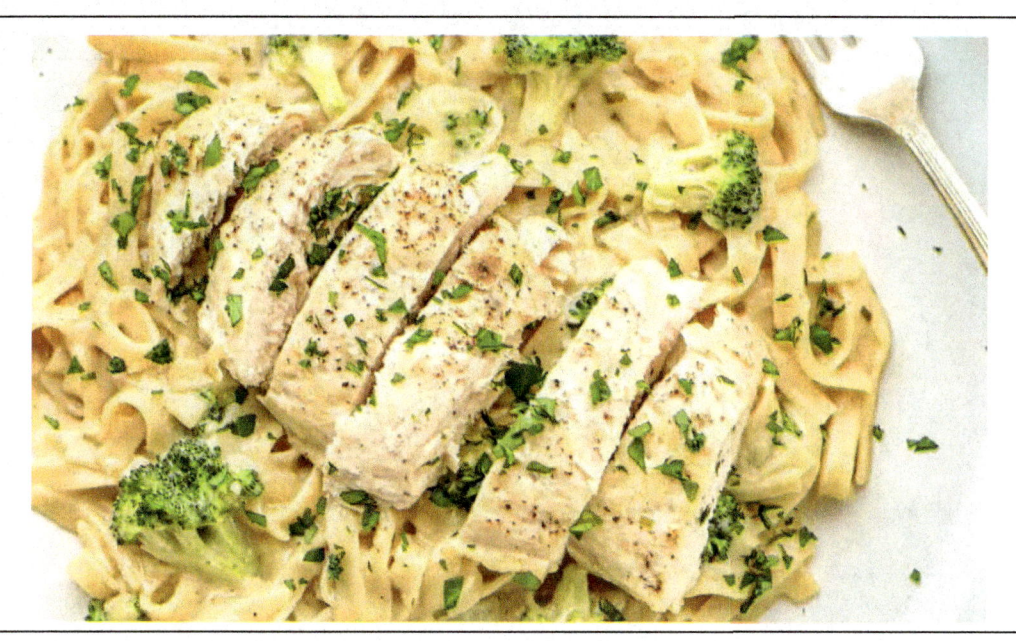

Vibe: Creamy Alfredo sauce served over gluten-free fettuccine pasta with grilled chicken, all made with low FODMAP ingredients

Ingredients

- 8 oz gluten-free fettuccine pasta
- 2 boneless, skinless chicken breasts, grilled and sliced
- 1 cup lactose-free cream
- 2 tablespoons butter
- 1/2 cup grated Parmesan cheese
- Salt and pepper to taste
- Chopped fresh parsley for garnish (optional)

Steps for Cooking:

1. Cook gluten-free fettuccine pasta according to package instructions and drain.
2. In a saucepan, melt butter over medium heat.
3. Add lactose-free cream and grated Parmesan cheese.
4. Stir continuously until the sauce thickens.
5. Season the sauce with salt and pepper to taste.
6. Serve the cooked pasta topped with grilled and sliced chicken.
7. Pour the creamy Alfredo sauce over the pasta and chicken.
8. Garnish with chopped fresh parsley if desired.

DAY 26

SPINACH AND CHEDDAR CHEESE MUFFINS (HOMEMADE WITH LOW FODMAP INGREDIENTS)

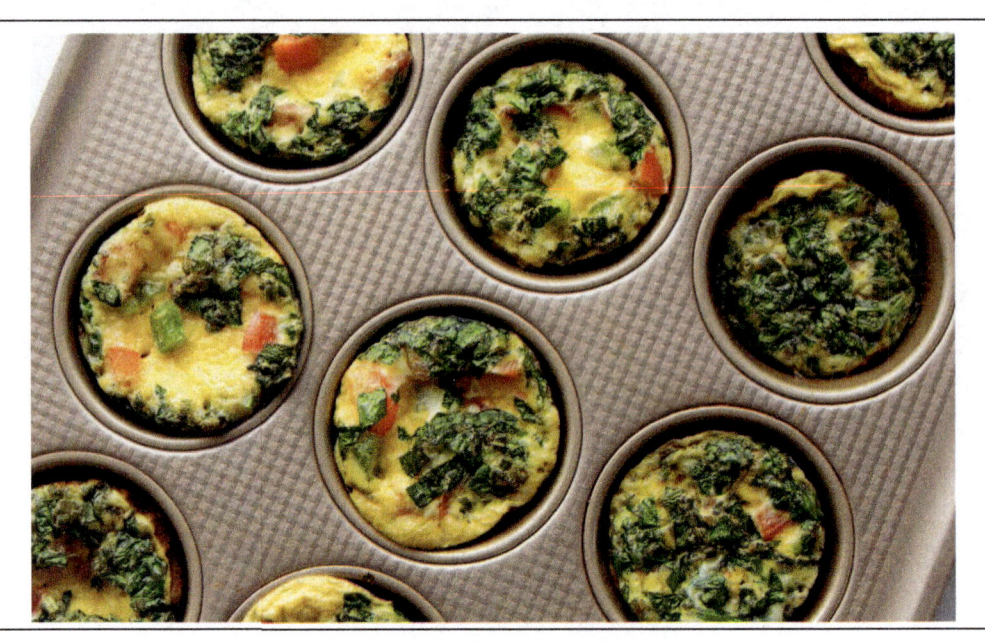

AVibe: Savory and cheesy muffins with the goodness of spinach.

Ingredients

- 1 cup fresh spinach leaves, chopped
- 1/2 cup grated cheddar cheese (check for FODMAP content)
- 1 cup gluten-free flour (check for FODMAP content)
- 2 teaspoons baking powder (check for FODMAP content)
- 1/2 teaspoon salt
- 1/2 cup lactose-free milk
- 1/4 cup olive oil
- 1 large egg

Steps for Cooking:

1. Preheat the oven to 375°F (190°C). Line a muffin tin with paper liners.
2. In a mixing bowl, combine chopped fresh spinach and grated cheddar cheese.
3. In a separate bowl, whisk together gluten-free flour, baking powder, and salt.
4. In another bowl, whisk together lactose-free milk, olive oil, and a large egg.
5. Combine the wet ingredients with the dry ingredients, then gently fold in the spinach and cheddar cheese mixture.
6. Fill each muffin cup about 2/3 full with the batter.
7. Bake for 18-20 minutes or until a toothpick inserted into a muffin comes out clean.
8. Allow the muffins to cool before serving.
9. Enjoy your homemade Low FODMAP spinach and cheddar cheese muffins.

STUFFED BELL PEPPERS WITH GROUND TURKEY AND RICE

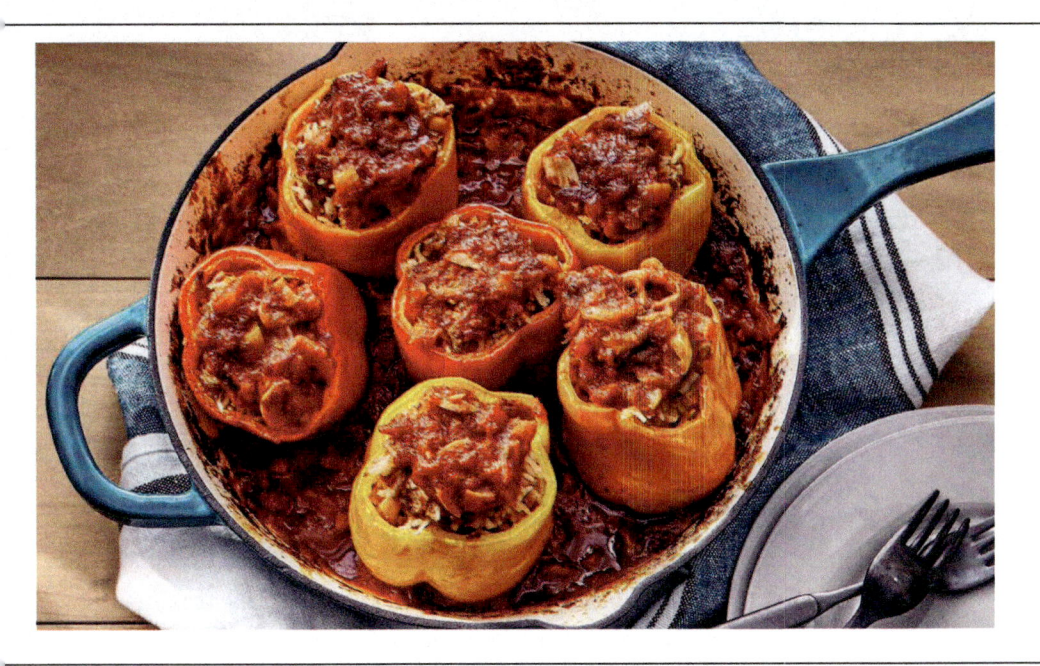

Vibe: Bell peppers stuffed with a flavorful mixture of ground turkey and rice.

Ingredients

- Bell peppers
- Ground turkey
- Cooked rice (check for FODMAP content)
- Olive oil, salt, and pepper for seasoning
- Tomato sauce (check for FODMAP content)

Steps for Cooking:

1. Preheat the oven to 375°F (190°C).
2. Cut the tops off the bell peppers and remove the seeds.
3. In a skillet, brown ground turkey in olive oil.
4. Add cooked rice and season with salt and pepper.
5. Stuff the bell peppers with the turkey and rice mixture.
6. Place the stuffed bell peppers in a baking dish and pour tomato sauce over them.
7. Bake for about 25-30 minutes or until the bell peppers are tender.

LOW FODMAP LAMB KEBABS (HOMEMADE WITH LOW FODMAP INGREDIENTS)

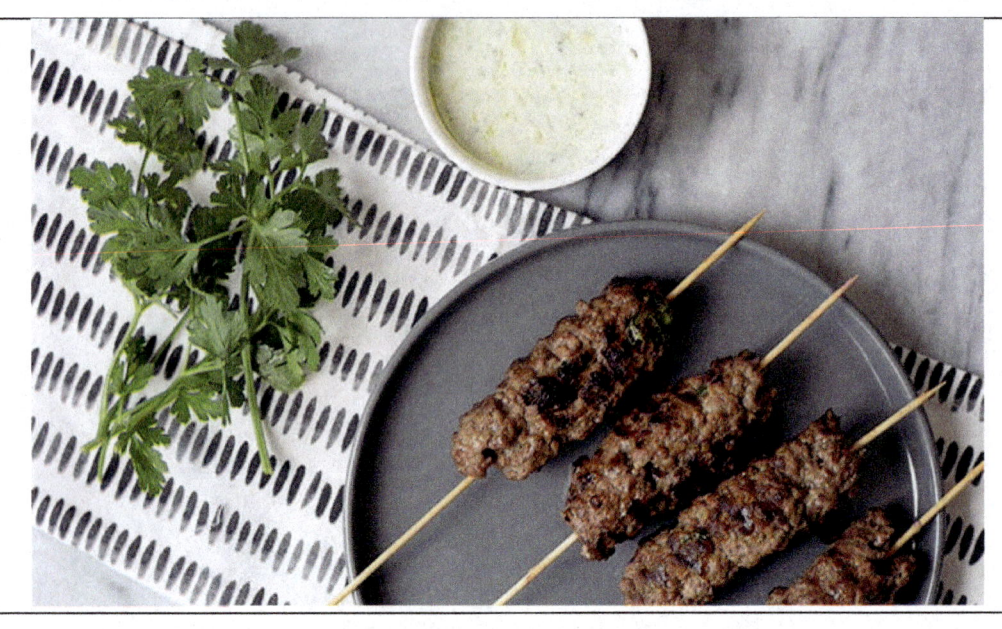

Vibe: Flavorful and tender lamb kebabs with a hint of minty freshness.

Ingredients

- 1 pound ground lamb
- 1/4 cup fresh mint leaves, chopped
- 1 tablespoon garlic-infused oil (discard garlic pieces)
- 1 teaspoon ground cumin
- 1 teaspoon ground coriander
- 1/2 teaspoon ground paprika (check for FODMAP content)
- Salt and pepper to taste
- Wooden skewers, soaked in water
- Fresh mint leaves for garnish
- Lactose-free yogurt (optional, for dipping)

Steps for Cooking:

1. In a mixing bowl, combine ground lamb, chopped fresh mint leaves, garlic-infused oil, ground cumin, ground coriander, ground paprika, salt, and pepper.
2. Mix the ingredients until well combined.
3. Divide the lamb mixture into portions and shape them into elongated kebabs around wooden skewers.
4. Preheat your grill to medium-high heat.
5. Grill the lamb kebabs for about 3-4 minutes per side or until they are cooked to your desired level of doneness.
6. Serve the Low FODMAP Lamb Kebabs garnished with fresh mint leaves and accompanied by lactose-free yogurt for dipping if desired.

DAY 27

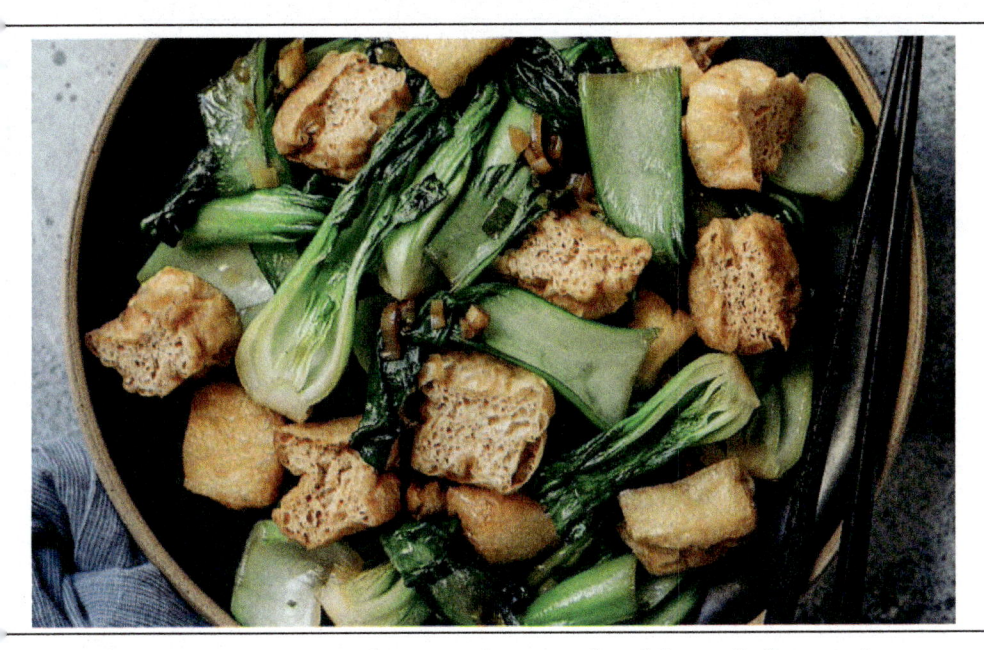

BREAKFAST STIR-FRY WITH TOFU, BOK CHOY, AND SESAME SEEDS

Vibe: A savory and protein-packed breakfast stir-fry with tofu, bok choy, and sesame seeds.

Ingredients

- 8 oz firm tofu, cubed
- 2 baby bok choy, chopped
- 1 tablespoon low-sodium soy sauce (check for FODMAP content)
- 1 teaspoon sesame oil
- Sesame seeds for garnish
- Olive oil for cooking

Steps for Cooking:

1. Heat a skillet or wok over medium heat with a drizzle of olive oil.
2. Add cubed tofu and stir-fry until lightly browned.
3. Add chopped bok choy and continue to stir-fry until bok choy is tender.
4. Drizzle low-sodium soy sauce and sesame oil over the stir-fry.
5. Toss to combine and heat through.

SAUTÉED KALE WITH BACON AND A SIDE OF GRILLED CHICKEN BREAST

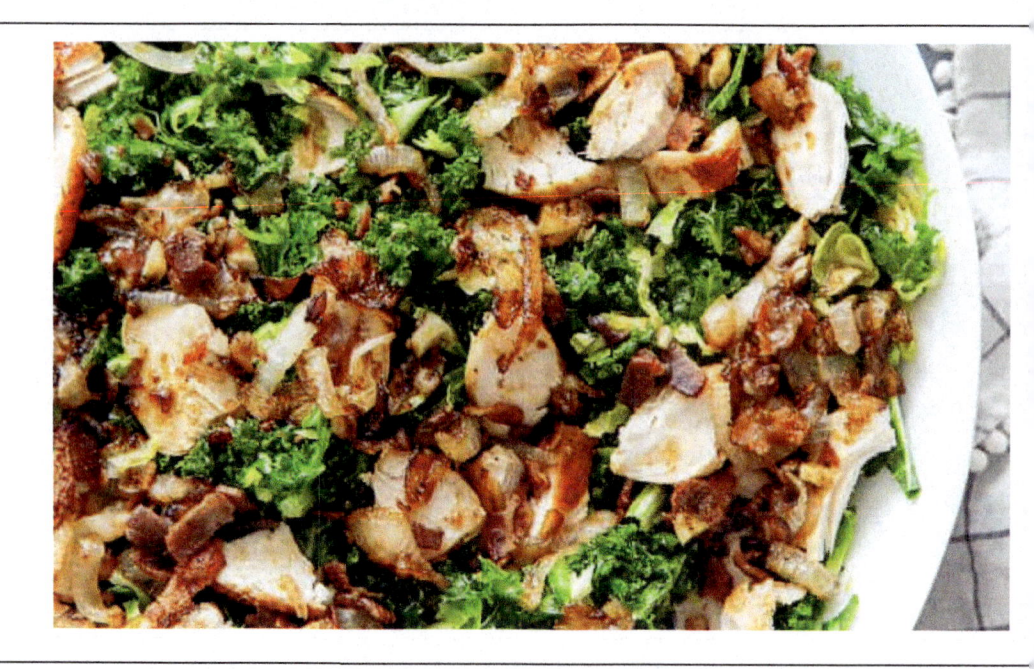

Vibe: Sautéed kale with crispy bacon, served with grilled chicken breast.

Ingredients

- Kale leaves, chopped
- Bacon strips (check for FODMAP content)
- Grilled chicken breast
- Olive oil, salt, and pepper for seasoning

Steps for Cooking:

1. In a skillet, cook bacon until crispy, then remove and crumble it.
2. In the same skillet, add olive oil and sauté chopped kale until wilted.
3. Season kale with salt and pepper.
4. Serve sautéed kale with crumbled bacon on top and grilled chicken breast on the side.
5. Enjoy your Low FODMAP sautéed kale with bacon and grilled chicken breast.

BAKED CHICKEN BREAST WITH ROASTED POTATOES AND CARROTS

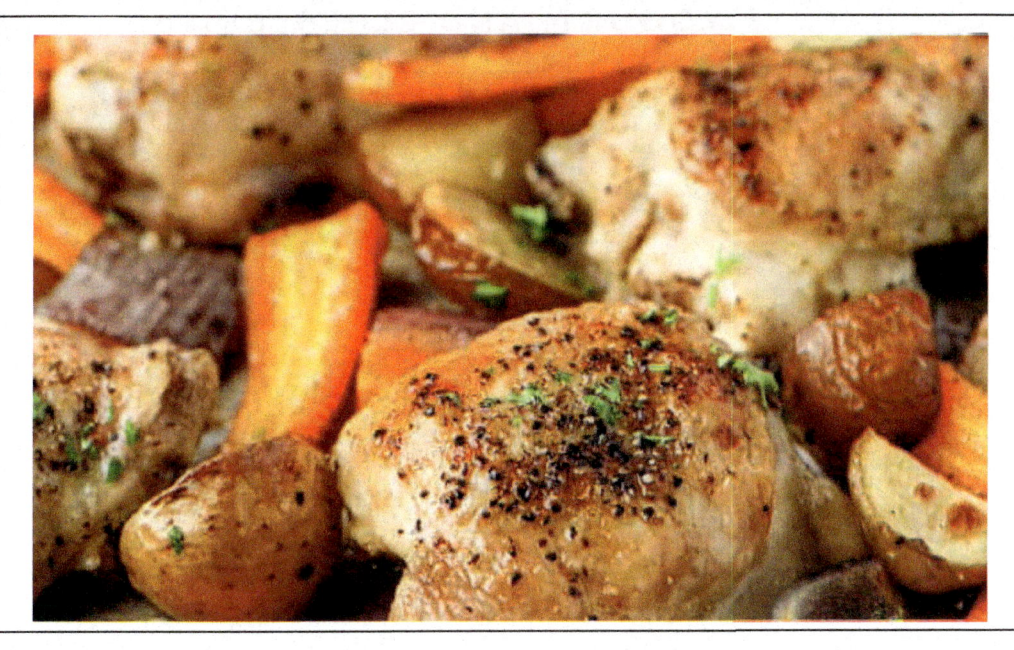

A homely and nourishing meal, combining the simplicity of baked chicken with the rustic charm of roasted potatoes and carrots.

Ingredients

- Chicken breast
- Potatoes (check for FODMAP content)
- Carrots
- Olive oil, salt, and pepper for seasoning

Steps for Cooking:

1. Preheat the oven to 375°F (190°C).
2. Season chicken breast with olive oil, salt, and pepper.
3. Bake chicken breast for about 20-25 minutes or until cooked through.
4. Roast potatoes and carrots until tender and slightly crispy.
5. Serve baked chicken breast with roasted potatoes and carrots.
6. Enjoy your Low FODMAP baked chicken breast with roasted potatoes and carrots.

DAY 28

SMOOTHIE WITH UNRIPE BANANA, LACTOSE-FREE YOGURT, AND BLUEBERRIES

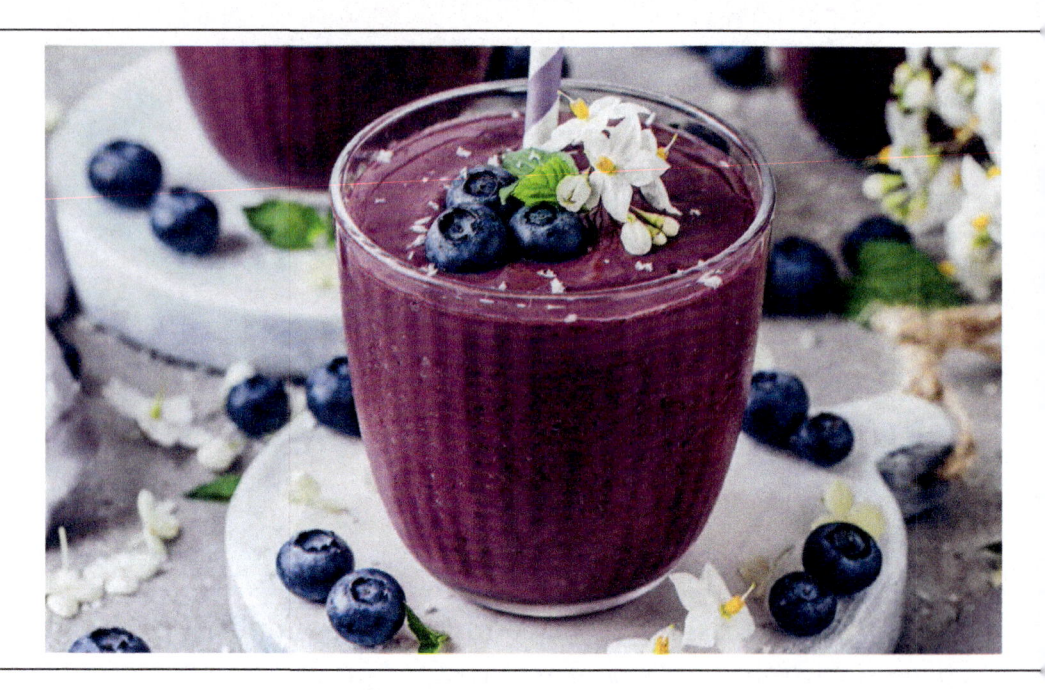

Vibe: A refreshing and Low FODMAP smoothie to start your day with a burst of energy.

Ingredients

- 1 unripe banana
- 1 cup lactose-free yogurt
- 1/2 cup blueberries
- Ice cubes (optional)
- A drizzle of maple syrup (optional for added sweetness)

Steps for Cooking:

1. Peel and slice the unripe banana.
2. In a blender, combine the banana slices, lactose-free yogurt, and blueberries.
3. Add ice cubes if you prefer a colder smoothie.
4. Blend until smooth and creamy.
5. Taste and add a drizzle of maple syrup if desired for extra sweetness.
6. Pour into a glass and enjoy your Low FODMAP smoothie.

LOW FODMAP SPAGHETTI WITH MEATBALLS
(HOMEMADE WITH LOW FODMAP INGREDIENTS)

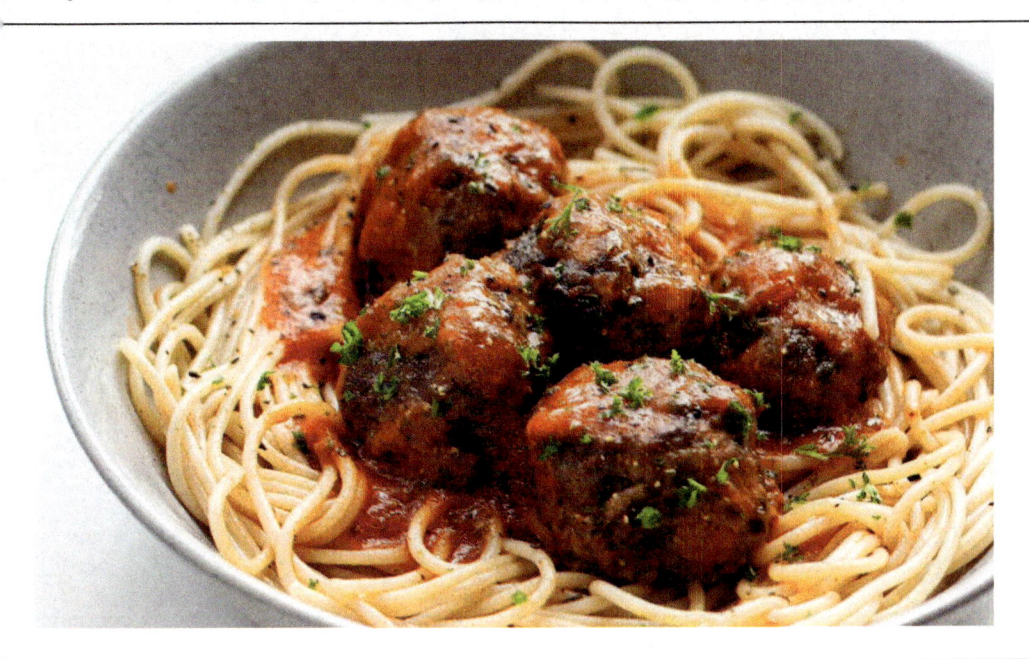

Vibe: Gluten-free spaghetti with homemade meatballs in a tomato sauce made with low FODMAP ingredients.

Ingredients

- For Meatballs:
- 1 pound ground beef or pork
- 1 egg
- Salt and pepper to taste
- For Tomato Sauce:
- 1 cup low FODMAP tomato sauce
- 1/2 cup canned diced tomatoes (check for FODMAP content)
- 1 teaspoon garlic-infused oil (discard garlic pieces)
- 1 teaspoon dried oregano
- Salt and pepper to taste
- Cooked gluten-free spaghetti

Steps for Cooking:

1. Lay out slices of turkey and Swiss cheese.
2. Place a slice of Swiss cheese on each slice of turkey.
3. Roll up the turkey and cheese slices and secure with toothpicks.
4. Serve with cherry tomatoes on the side.
5. Enjoy your Low FODMAP turkey and Swiss cheese roll-ups.

TURKEY AND CHEDDAR CHEESE STUFFED BELL PEPPERS

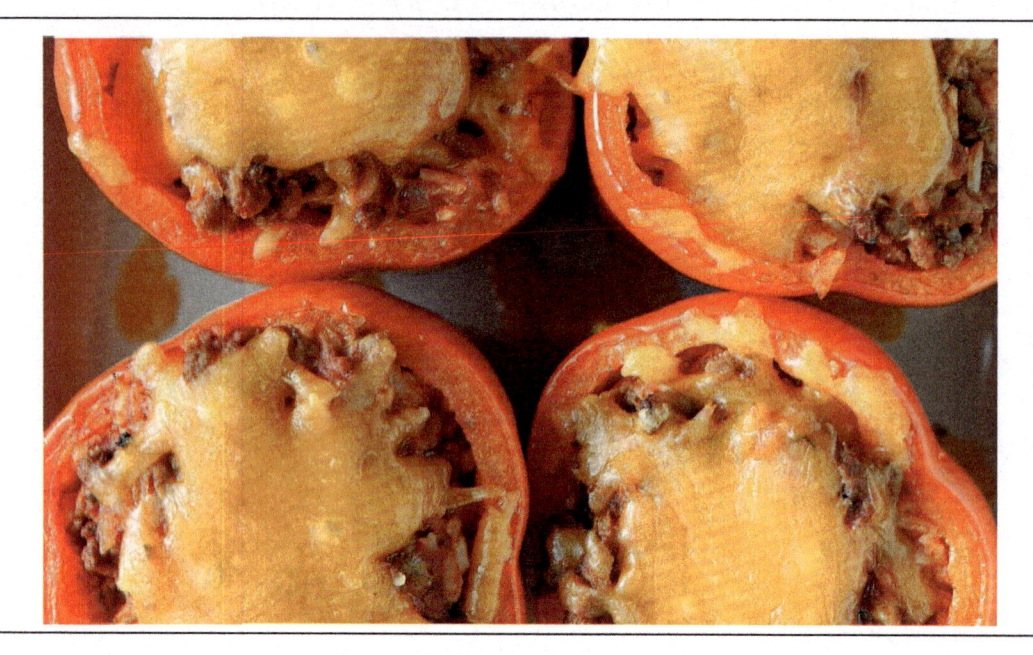

A cheesy and satisfying dish, where bell peppers are generously filled with a flavorful mixture of turkey and cheddar, creating a comforting meal.

Ingredients

- Bell peppers
- Ground turkey
- Cheddar cheese (if tolerated)
- Olive oil, salt, and pepper for seasoning

Steps for Cooking:

1. Preheat the oven to 375°F (190°C).
2. Cut the tops off the bell peppers and remove the seeds.
3. In a skillet, cook ground turkey in olive oil until browned.
4. Stir in cheddar cheese (if tolerated) until melted and combined.
5. Season with salt and pepper.
6. Stuff the bell peppers with the turkey and cheddar cheese mixture.
7. Place the stuffed bell peppers in a baking dish.
8. Bake for about 25-30 minutes or until the bell peppers are tender.
9. Enjoy your Low FODMAP turkey and cheddar cheese stuffed bell peppers.

After completing Week 4, it's important to reflect on how your body has responded to the dietary changes. Use the following scale to rate your experiences in various aspects of your health and well-being. Rate each category from 1 to 10 (where 1 is 'no improvement' and 10 is 'significant improvement').

1. Digestive Comfort
- Question: How would you rate the overall comfort of your digestive system this week?
- Rating (1-10): _ _ _ _ _

2. Energy Levels
- Question: How do you feel about your energy levels after following the meal plan for a week?
- Rating (1-10): _ _ _ _ _

3. Sleep Quality
- Question: Have you noticed any changes in the quality of your sleep?
- Rating (1-10): _ _ _ _ _

4. Mood and Mental Clarity
- Question: How has your mood and mental clarity been affected by the dietary changes?
- Rating (1-10): _ _ _ _ _

5. Physical Comfort and Pain Levels
- Question: If you previously experienced any physical discomfort or pain, have you noticed any changes in its intensity or frequency?
- Rating (1-10): _ _ _ _ _

6. Skin Health
- Question: Have there been any noticeable changes in your skin health/appearance?
- Rating (1-10): _ _ _ _ _

7. Cravings and Appetite Control
- Question: How would you rate your control over cravings and appetite this week?
- Rating (1-10): _ _ _ _ _

8. Overall Well-being
- Question: Considering all factors, how would you rate your overall well-being after Week 1?
- Rating (1-10): _ _ _ _ _

FOR SPECIAL *notes*

COMPLETION OF YOUR FODMAP JOURNEY - A HEARTFELT THANK YOU

I want to extend a heartfelt thank you for your dedication and perseverance. Your journey doesn't end here; it's a continual path of discovery and adjustment. Remember, the insights and habits you've developed over these weeks are tools that will empower you to maintain a happy and healthy gut for years to come. Congratulations on this remarkable achievement! Remember to to do your FODMAP Journey Progress Table.

FODMAP JOURNEY PROGRESS TABLE

This table will allow you to visually compare your experiences across various health aspects over the four weeks of the diet. Here's a structure you can follow

DATE:	SLEEP	WEIGHT
	1 2 3 4 5 6 7 8 9 10	

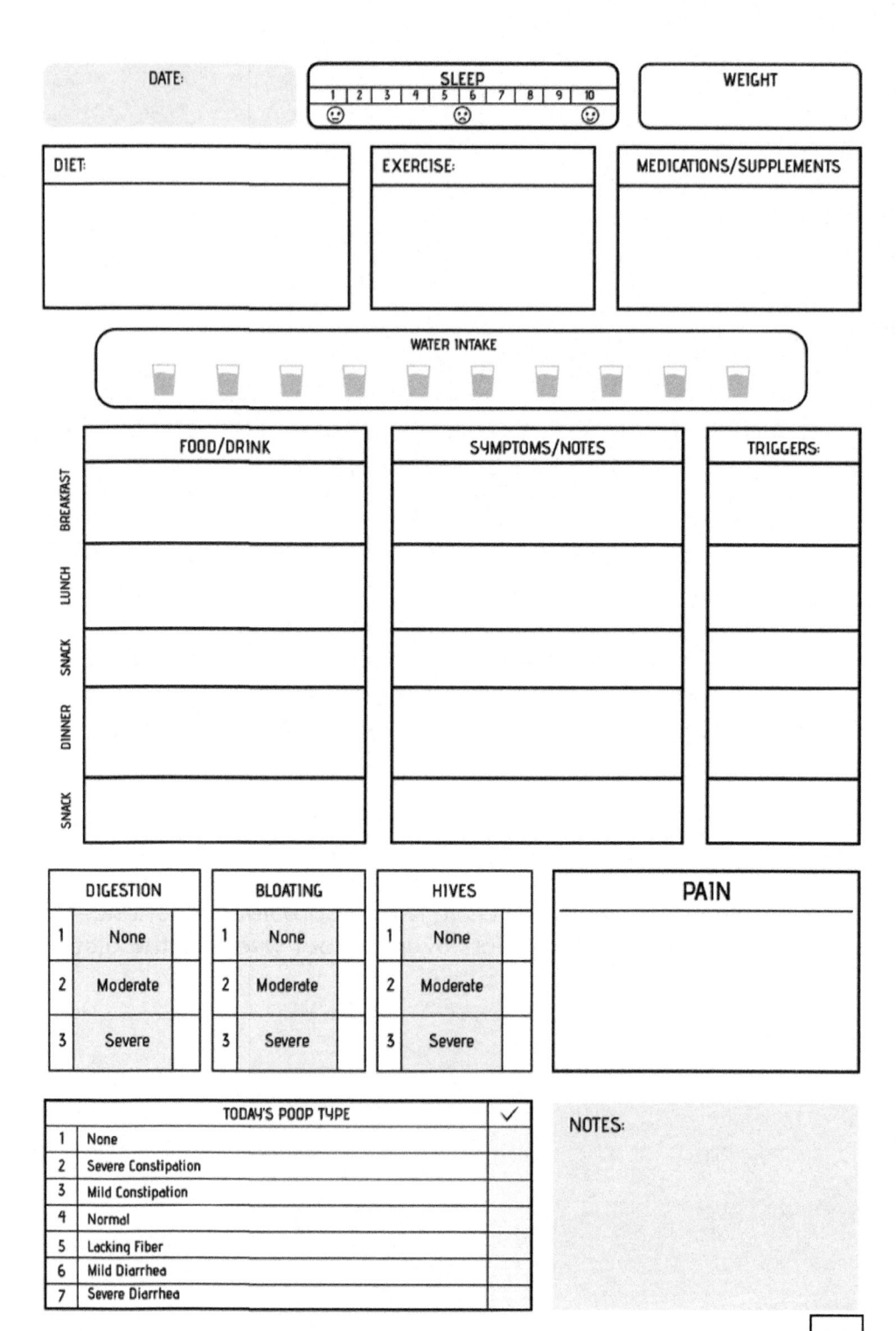

DIET:	EXERCISE:	MEDICATIONS/SUPPLEMENTS

WATER INTAKE

	FOOD/DRINK	SYMPTOMS/NOTES	TRIGGERS:
BREAKFAST			
LUNCH			
SNACK			
DINNER			
SNACK			

DIGESTION		BLOATING		HIVES	
1	None	1	None	1	None
2	Moderate	2	Moderate	2	Moderate
3	Severe	3	Severe	3	Severe

PAIN

	TODAY'S POOP TYPE	✓
1	None	
2	Severe Constipation	
3	Mild Constipation	
4	Normal	
5	Lacking Fiber	
6	Mild Diarrhea	
7	Severe Diarrhea	

NOTES:

DATE:

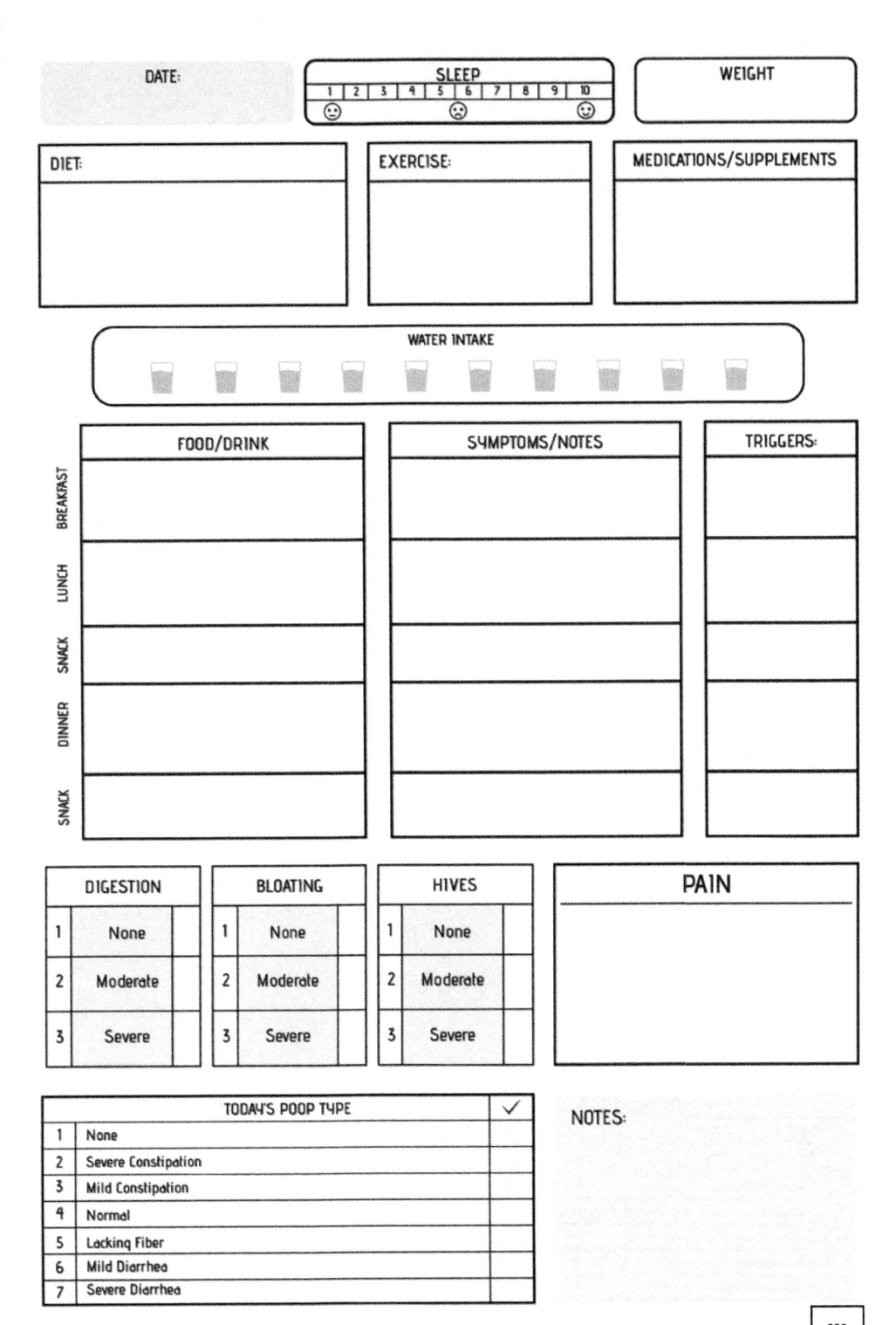

SLEEP 1 2 3 4 5 6 7 8 9 10

WEIGHT

DIET:

EXERCISE:

MEDICATIONS/SUPPLEMENTS

WATER INTAKE

	FOOD/DRINK	SYMPTOMS/NOTES	TRIGGERS:
BREAKFAST			
LUNCH			
SNACK			
DINNER			
SNACK			

DIGESTION			BLOATING			HIVES	
1	None		1	None		1	None
2	Moderate		2	Moderate		2	Moderate
3	Severe		3	Severe		3	Severe

PAIN

	TODAY'S POOP TYPE	✓
1	None	
2	Severe Constipation	
3	Mild Constipation	
4	Normal	
5	Lacking Fiber	
6	Mild Diarrhea	
7	Severe Diarrhea	

NOTES:

DATE:

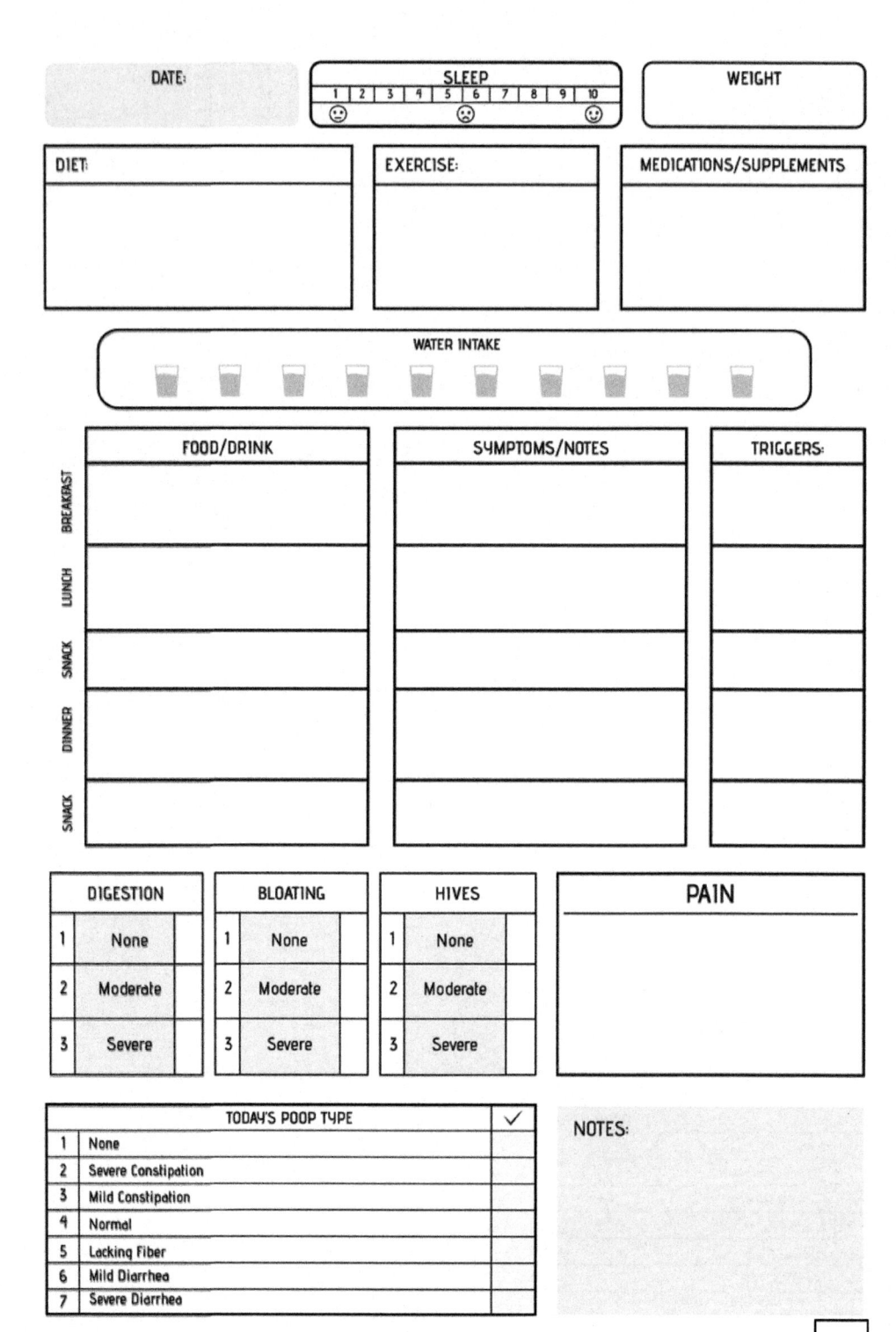

SLEEP
1	2	3	4	5	6	7	8	9	10

WEIGHT

DIET:

EXERCISE:

MEDICATIONS/SUPPLEMENTS

WATER INTAKE

	FOOD/DRINK	SYMPTOMS/NOTES	TRIGGERS:
BREAKFAST			
LUNCH			
SNACK			
DINNER			
SNACK			

DIGESTION
1	None
2	Moderate
3	Severe

BLOATING
1	None
2	Moderate
3	Severe

HIVES
1	None
2	Moderate
3	Severe

PAIN

TODAY'S POOP TYPE ✓
1	None
2	Severe Constipation
3	Mild Constipation
4	Normal
5	Lacking Fiber
6	Mild Diarrhea
7	Severe Diarrhea

NOTES:

DATE:

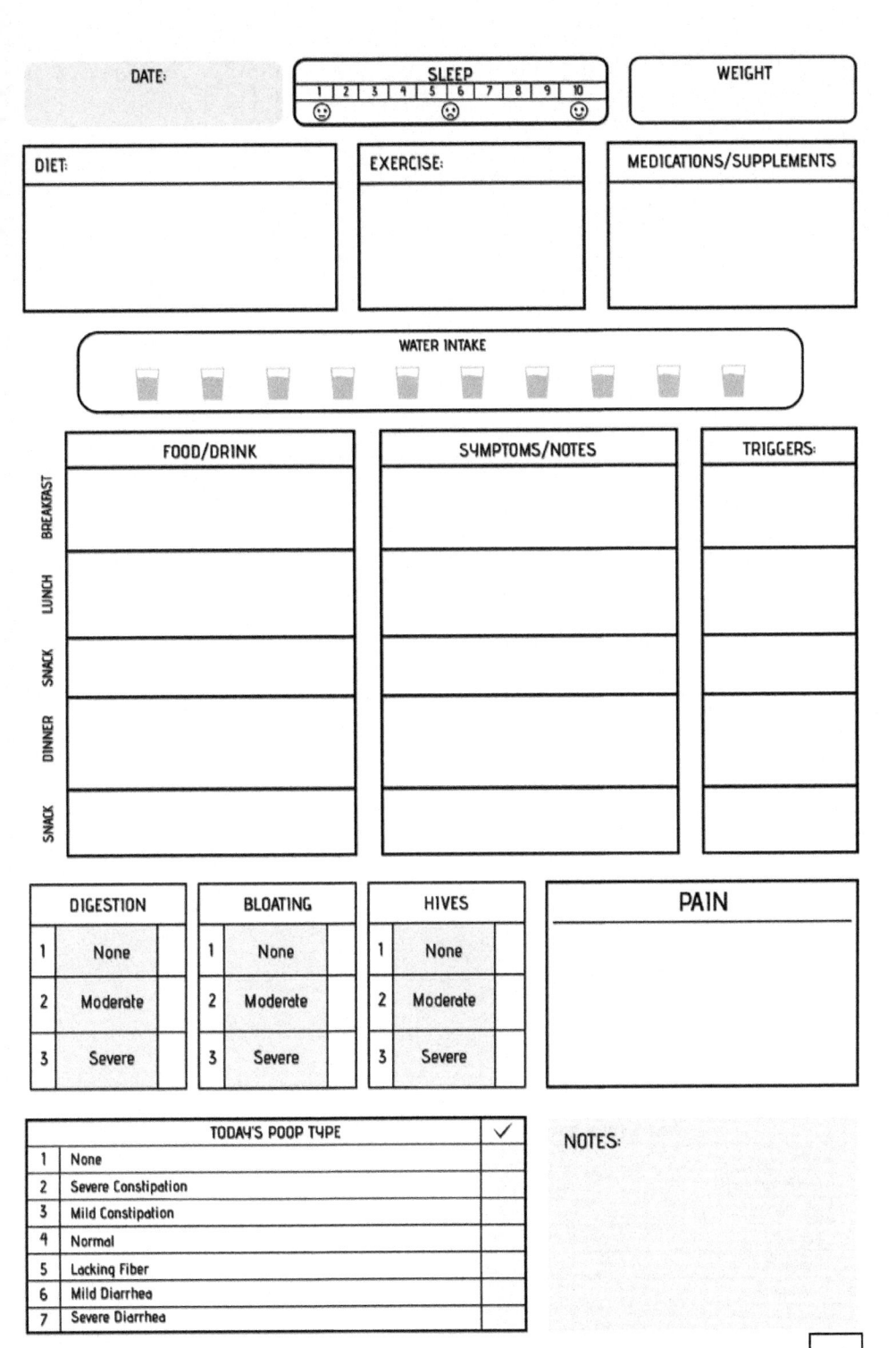

SLEEP
| 1 | 2 | 3 | 4 | 5 | 6 | 7 | 8 | 9 | 10 |

WEIGHT

DIET:

EXERCISE:

MEDICATIONS/SUPPLEMENTS

WATER INTAKE

	FOOD/DRINK	SYMPTOMS/NOTES	TRIGGERS:
BREAKFAST			
LUNCH			
SNACK			
DINNER			
SNACK			

DIGESTION		BLOATING		HIVES	
1	None	1	None	1	None
2	Moderate	2	Moderate	2	Moderate
3	Severe	3	Severe	3	Severe

PAIN

	TODAY'S POOP TYPE	✓
1	None	
2	Severe Constipation	
3	Mild Constipation	
4	Normal	
5	Lacking Fiber	
6	Mild Diarrhea	
7	Severe Diarrhea	

NOTES:

DATE:

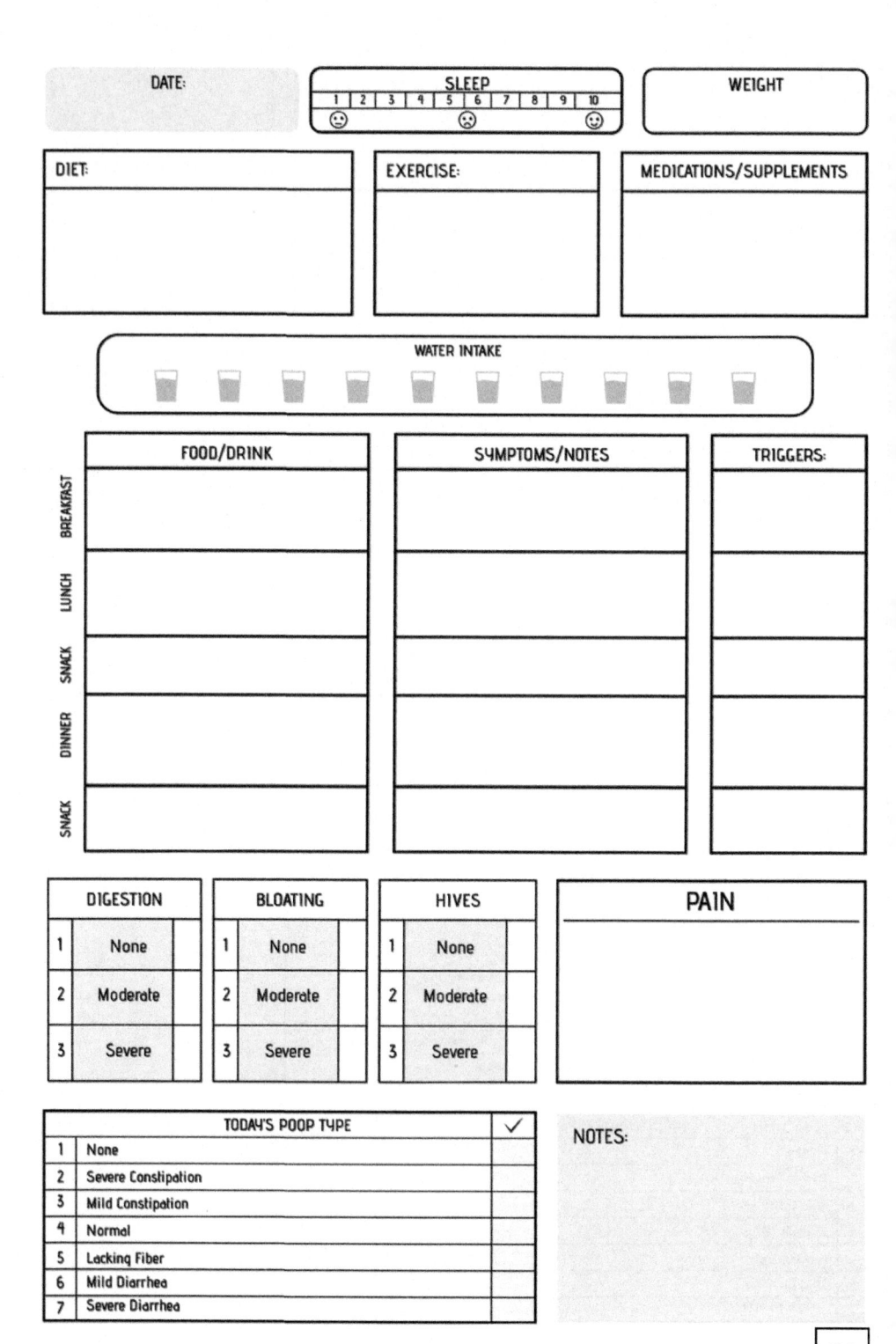

SLEEP
1	2	3	4	5	6	7	8	9	10

WEIGHT

DIET:

EXERCISE:

MEDICATIONS/SUPPLEMENTS

WATER INTAKE

	FOOD/DRINK	SYMPTOMS/NOTES	TRIGGERS:
BREAKFAST			
LUNCH			
SNACK			
DINNER			
SNACK			

DIGESTION
1	None
2	Moderate
3	Severe

BLOATING
1	None
2	Moderate
3	Severe

HIVES
1	None
2	Moderate
3	Severe

PAIN

TODAY'S POOP TYPE
1	None	
2	Severe Constipation	
3	Mild Constipation	
4	Normal	
5	Lacking Fiber	
6	Mild Diarrhea	
7	Severe Diarrhea	

NOTES:

DATE:

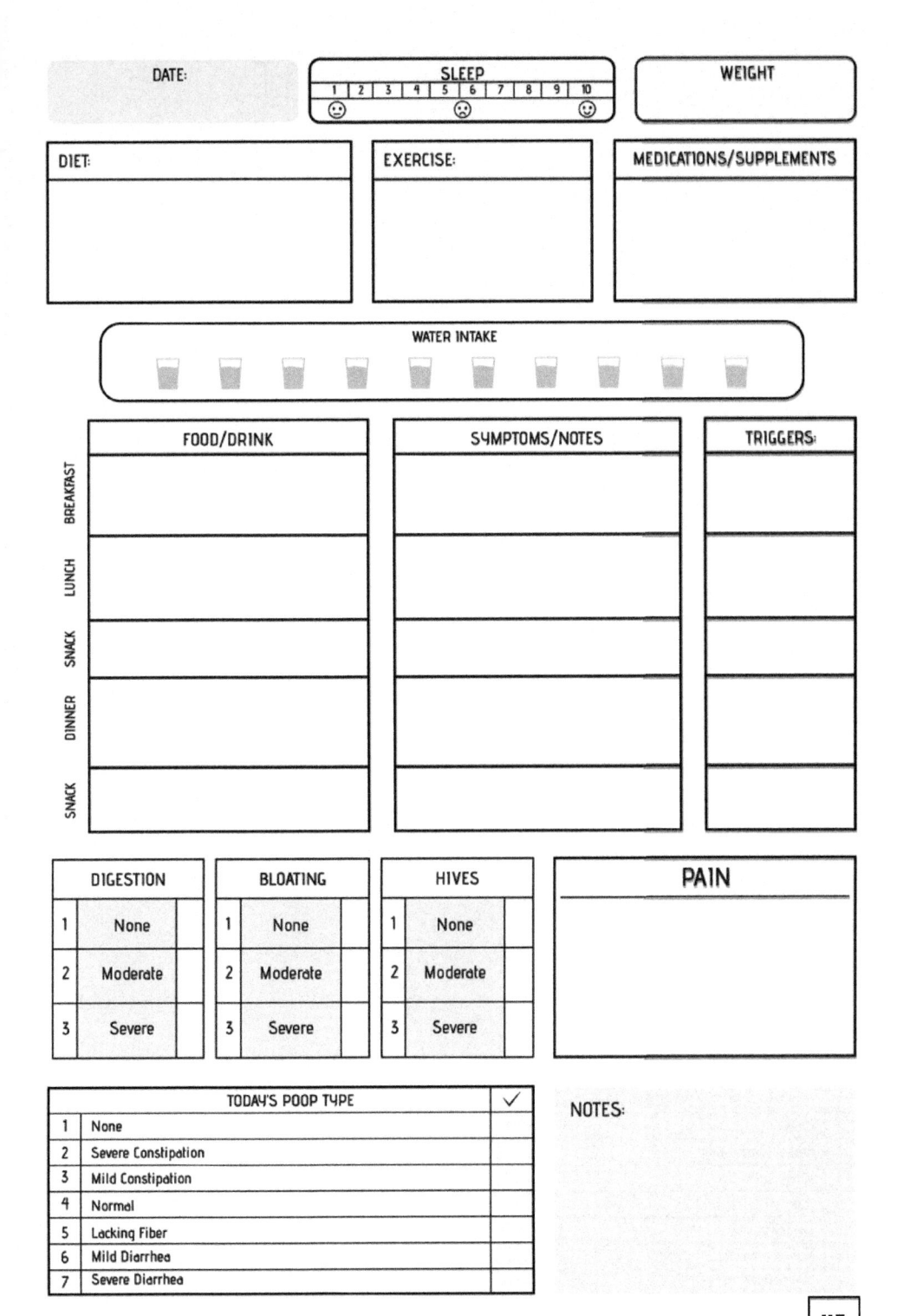

SLEEP
1	2	3	4	5	6	7	8	9	10

WEIGHT

DIET:

EXERCISE:

MEDICATIONS/SUPPLEMENTS

WATER INTAKE

FOOD/DRINK	SYMPTOMS/NOTES	TRIGGERS:
BREAKFAST		
LUNCH		
SNACK		
DINNER		
SNACK		

DIGESTION
1	None
2	Moderate
3	Severe

BLOATING
1	None
2	Moderate
3	Severe

HIVES
1	None
2	Moderate
3	Severe

PAIN

	TODAY'S POOP TYPE	✓
1	None	
2	Severe Constipation	
3	Mild Constipation	
4	Normal	
5	Lacking Fiber	
6	Mild Diarrhea	
7	Severe Diarrhea	

NOTES:

DATE:

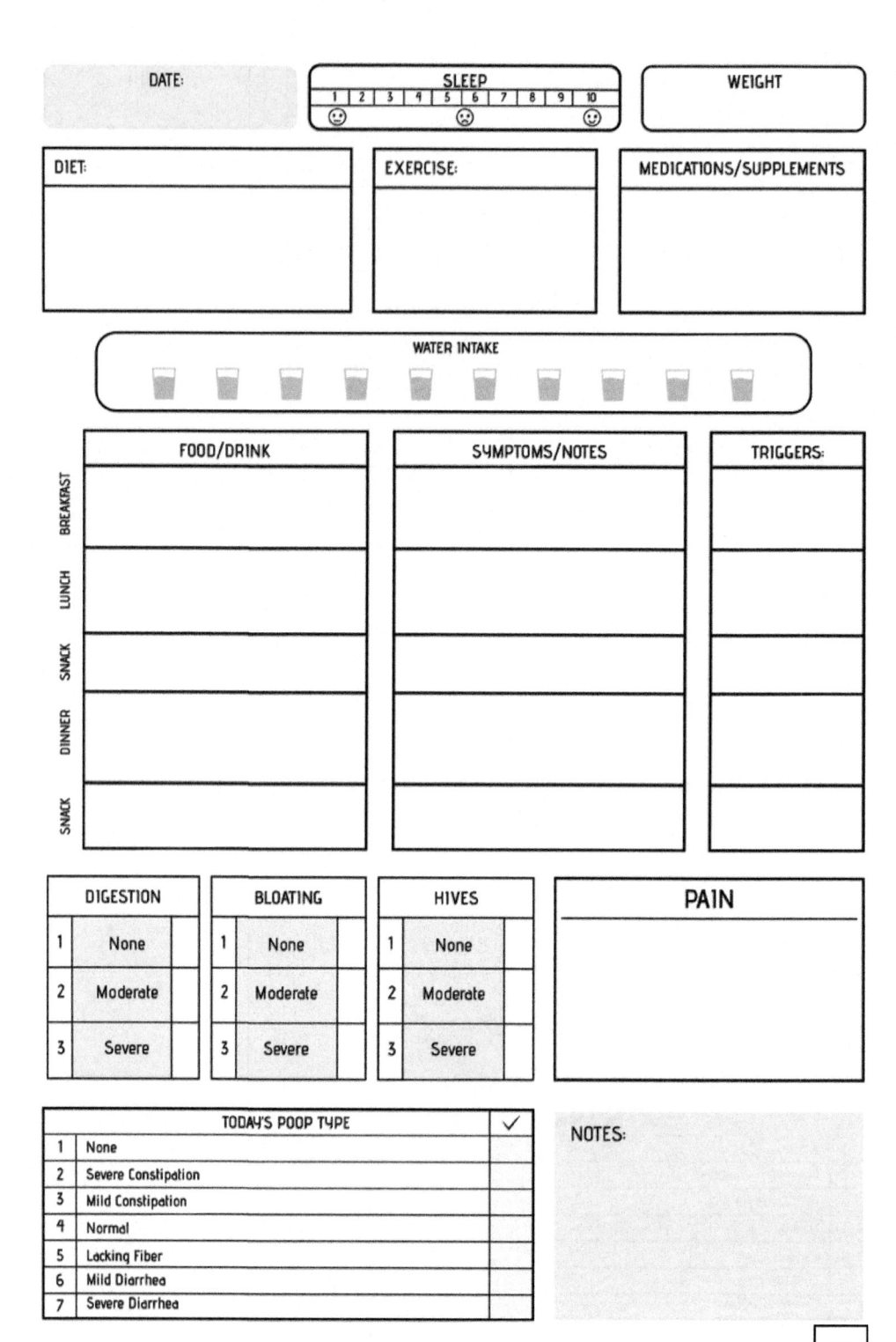

SLEEP
1	2	3	4	5	6	7	8	9	10

WEIGHT

DIET:

EXERCISE:

MEDICATIONS/SUPPLEMENTS

WATER INTAKE

	FOOD/DRINK	SYMPTOMS/NOTES	TRIGGERS:
BREAKFAST			
LUNCH			
SNACK			
DINNER			
SNACK			

DIGESTION
1	None
2	Moderate
3	Severe

BLOATING
1	None
2	Moderate
3	Severe

HIVES
1	None
2	Moderate
3	Severe

PAIN

TODAY'S POOP TYPE ✓
1	None
2	Severe Constipation
3	Mild Constipation
4	Normal
5	Lacking Fiber
6	Mild Diarrhea
7	Severe Diarrhea

NOTES:

DATE:

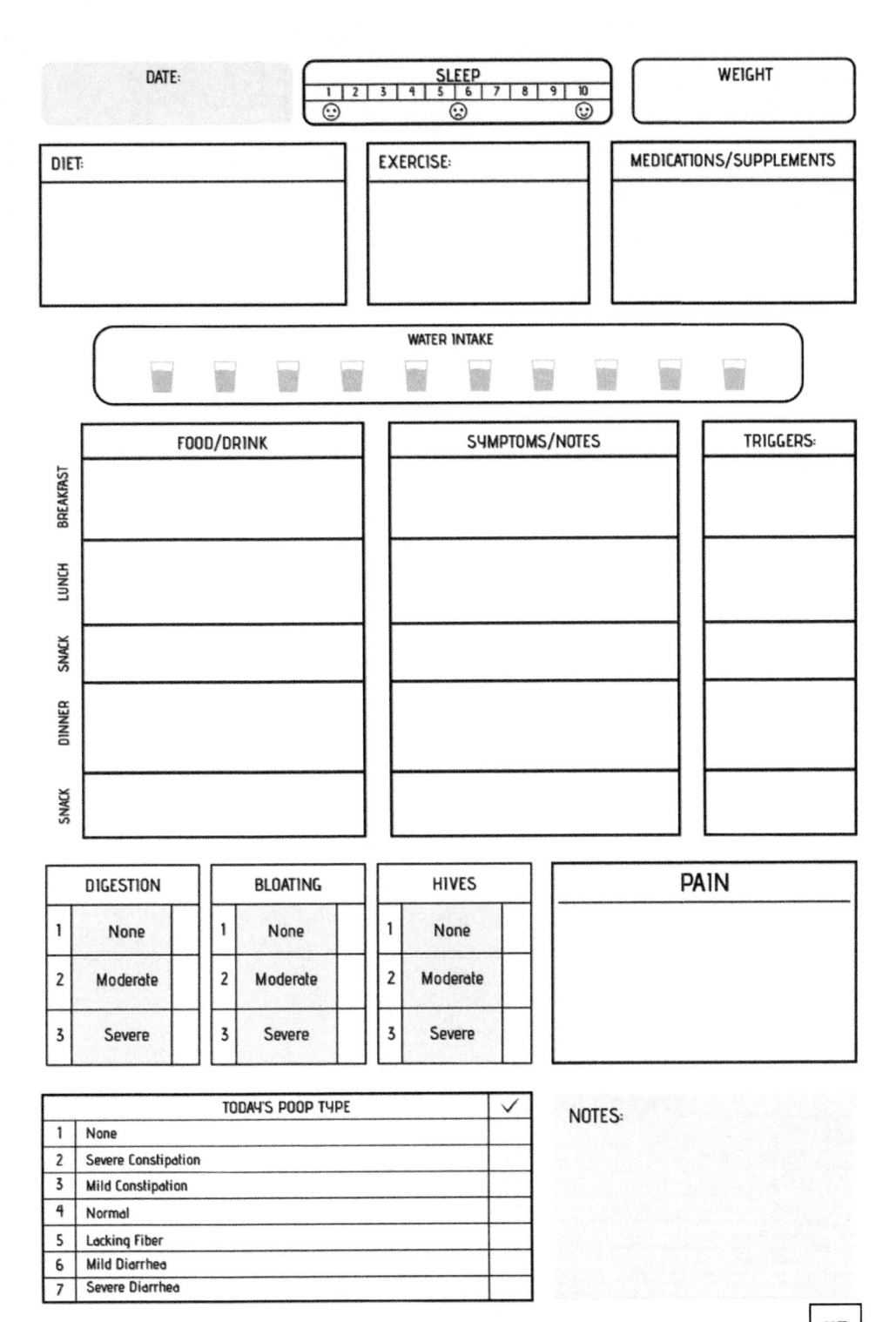

SLEEP
1	2	3	4	5	6	7	8	9	10

WEIGHT

DIET:

EXERCISE:

MEDICATIONS/SUPPLEMENTS

WATER INTAKE

	FOOD/DRINK	SYMPTOMS/NOTES	TRIGGERS:
BREAKFAST			
LUNCH			
SNACK			
DINNER			
SNACK			

DIGESTION
1	None
2	Moderate
3	Severe

BLOATING
1	None
2	Moderate
3	Severe

HIVES
1	None
2	Moderate
3	Severe

PAIN

TODAY'S POOP TYPE ✓
1	None	
2	Severe Constipation	
3	Mild Constipation	
4	Normal	
5	Lacking Fiber	
6	Mild Diarrhea	
7	Severe Diarrhea	

NOTES:

DATE:	SLEEP	WEIGHT

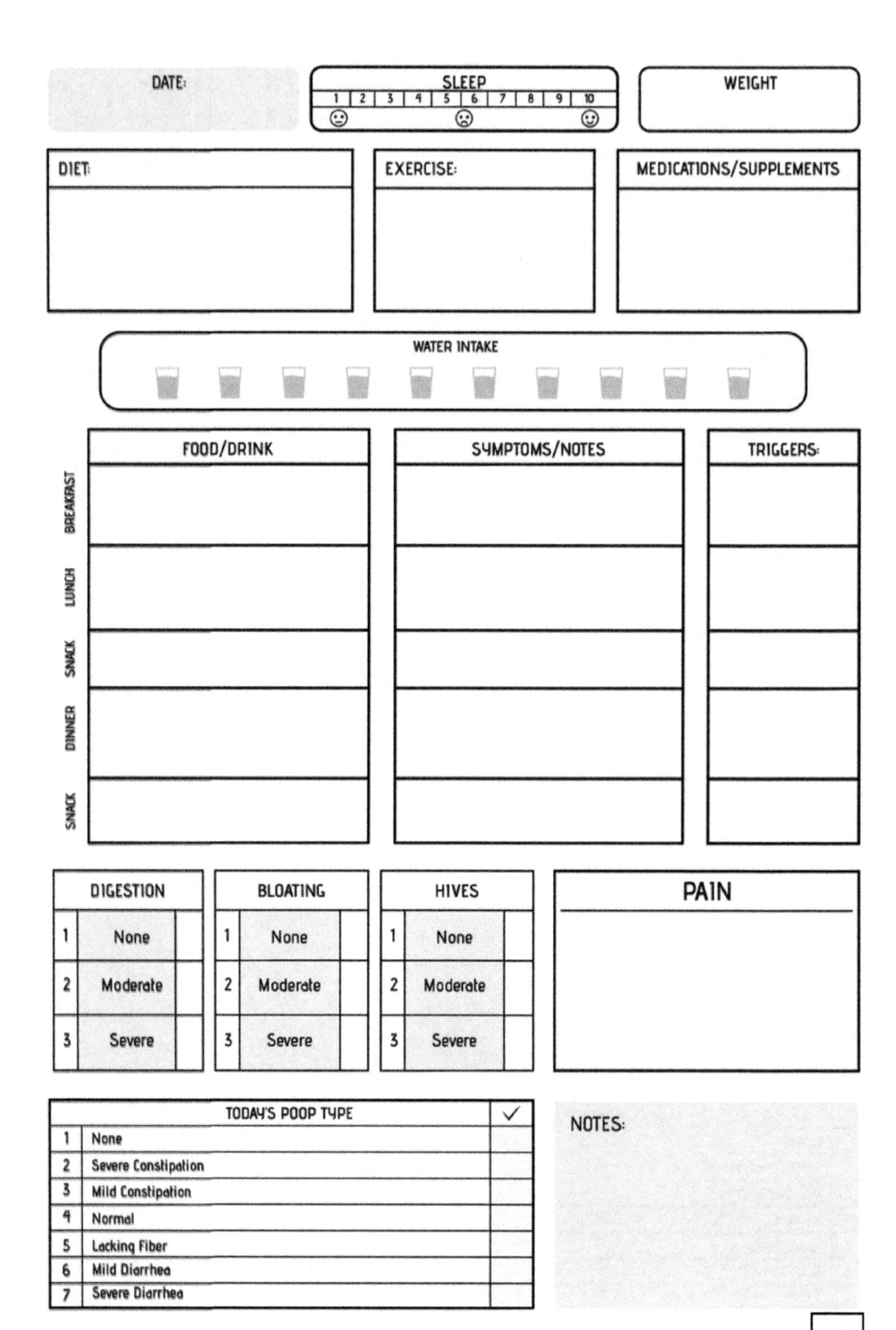

SLEEP: 1 2 3 4 5 6 7 8 9 10

DIET:	EXERCISE:	MEDICATIONS/SUPPLEMENTS

WATER INTAKE

	FOOD/DRINK	SYMPTOMS/NOTES	TRIGGERS:
BREAKFAST			
LUNCH			
SNACK			
DINNER			
SNACK			

	DIGESTION
1	None
2	Moderate
3	Severe

	BLOATING
1	None
2	Moderate
3	Severe

	HIVES
1	None
2	Moderate
3	Severe

PAIN

	TODAY'S POOP TYPE	✓
1	None	
2	Severe Constipation	
3	Mild Constipation	
4	Normal	
5	Lacking Fiber	
6	Mild Diarrhea	
7	Severe Diarrhea	

NOTES:

DATE:

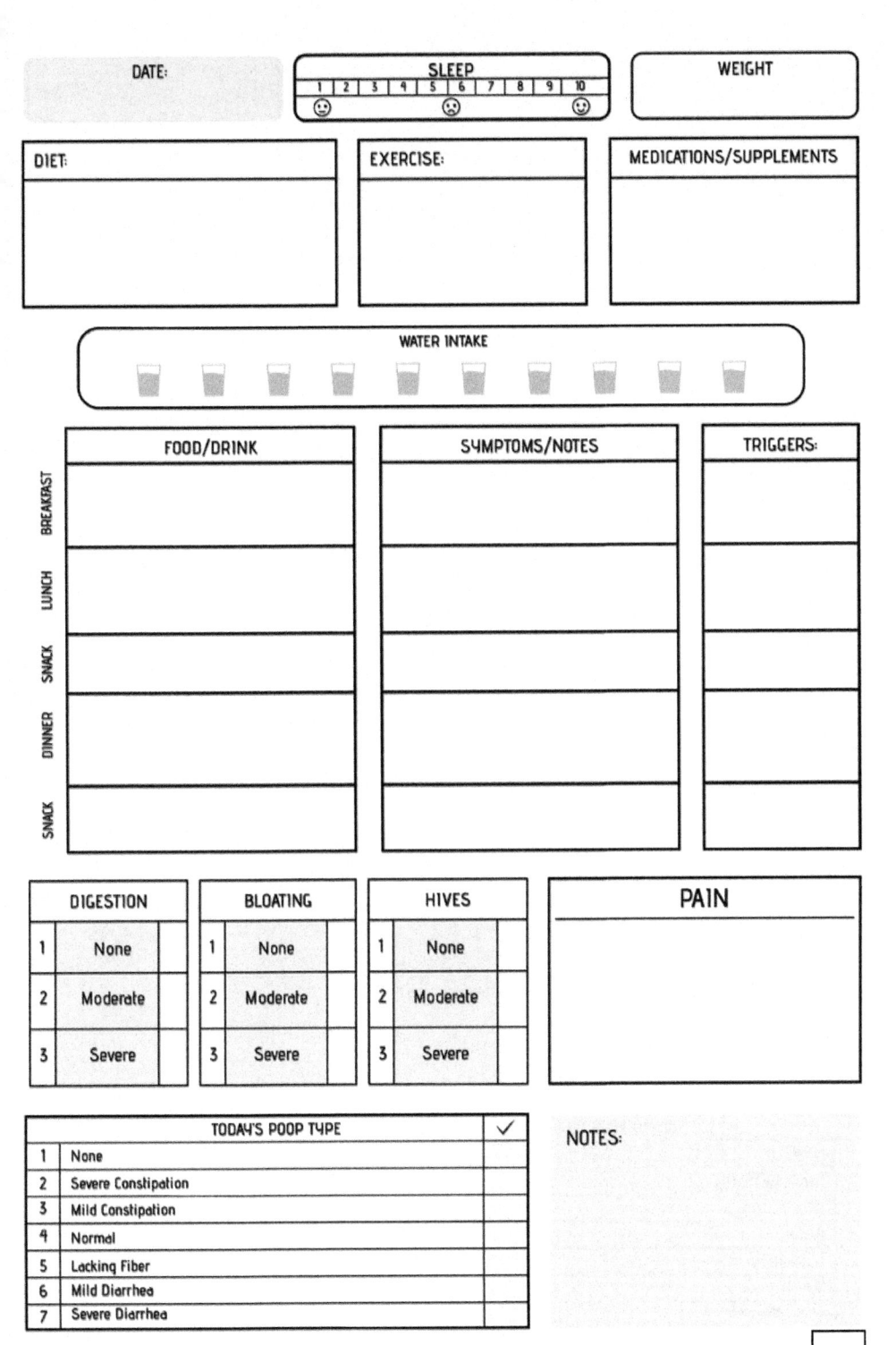

SLEEP
1	2	3	4	5	6	7	8	9	10

WEIGHT

DIET:

EXERCISE:

MEDICATIONS/SUPPLEMENTS

WATER INTAKE

	FOOD/DRINK	SYMPTOMS/NOTES	TRIGGERS:
BREAKFAST			
LUNCH			
SNACK			
DINNER			
SNACK			

DIGESTION
1	None
2	Moderate
3	Severe

BLOATING
1	None
2	Moderate
3	Severe

HIVES
1	None
2	Moderate
3	Severe

PAIN

TODAY'S POOP TYPE
		✓
1	None	
2	Severe Constipation	
3	Mild Constipation	
4	Normal	
5	Lacking Fiber	
6	Mild Diarrhea	
7	Severe Diarrhea	

NOTES:

DATE:

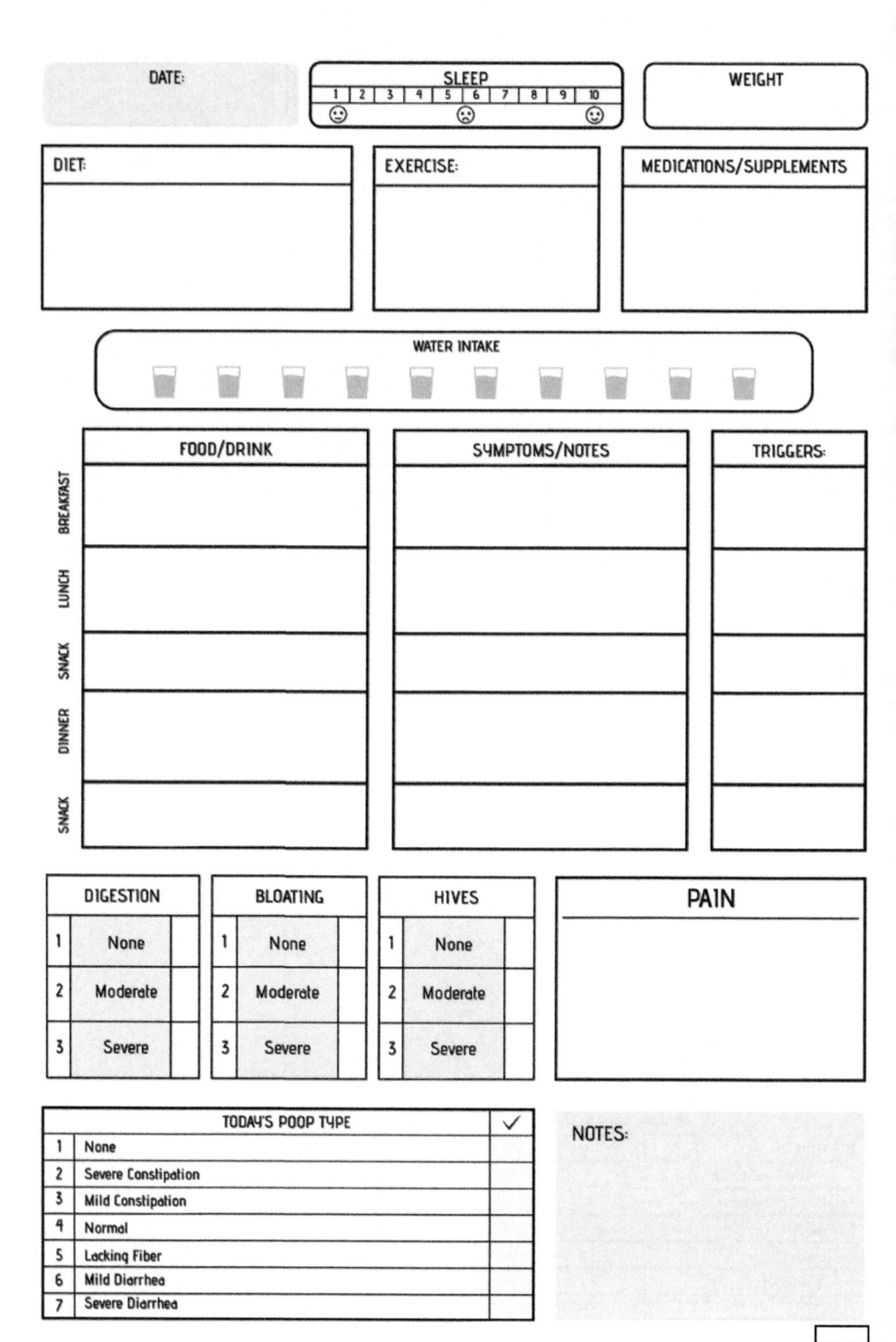

SLEEP
| 1 | 2 | 3 | 4 | 5 | 6 | 7 | 8 | 9 | 10 |

WEIGHT

DIET:

EXERCISE:

MEDICATIONS/SUPPLEMENTS

WATER INTAKE

	FOOD/DRINK	SYMPTOMS/NOTES	TRIGGERS:
BREAKFAST			
LUNCH			
SNACK			
DINNER			
SNACK			

DIGESTION
1	None
2	Moderate
3	Severe

BLOATING
1	None
2	Moderate
3	Severe

HIVES
1	None
2	Moderate
3	Severe

PAIN

	TODAY'S POOP TYPE	✓
1	None	
2	Severe Constipation	
3	Mild Constipation	
4	Normal	
5	Lacking Fiber	
6	Mild Diarrhea	
7	Severe Diarrhea	

NOTES:

DATE:

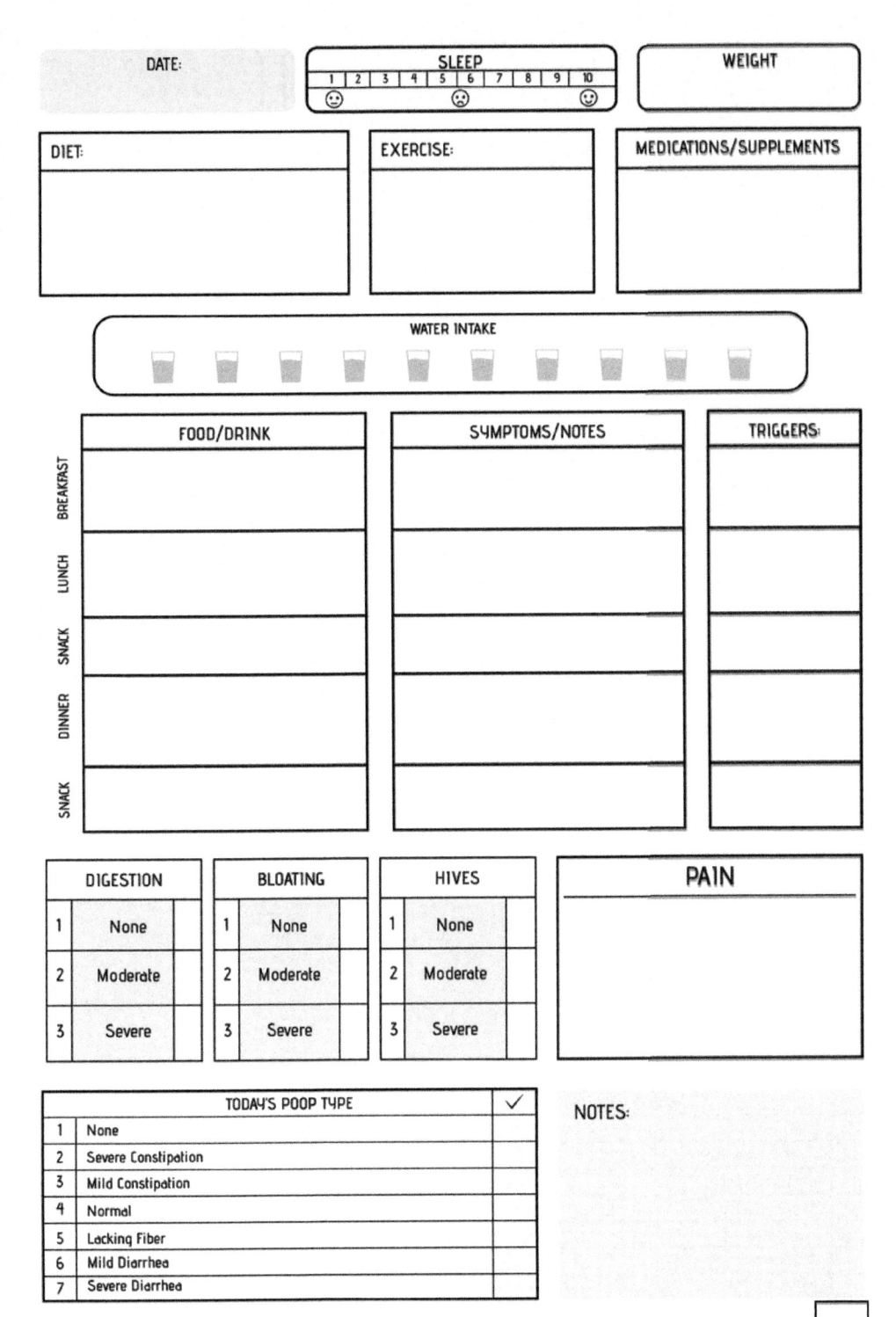

SLEEP
1	2	3	4	5	6	7	8	9	10
☹				☹					☺

WEIGHT

DIET:

EXERCISE:

MEDICATIONS/SUPPLEMENTS

WATER INTAKE

	FOOD/DRINK	SYMPTOMS/NOTES	TRIGGERS:
BREAKFAST			
LUNCH			
SNACK			
DINNER			
SNACK			

DIGESTION
1	None
2	Moderate
3	Severe

BLOATING
1	None
2	Moderate
3	Severe

HIVES
1	None
2	Moderate
3	Severe

PAIN

	TODAY'S POOP TYPE	✓
1	None	
2	Severe Constipation	
3	Mild Constipation	
4	Normal	
5	Lacking Fiber	
6	Mild Diarrhea	
7	Severe Diarrhea	

NOTES:

DATE: SLEEP   WEIGHT

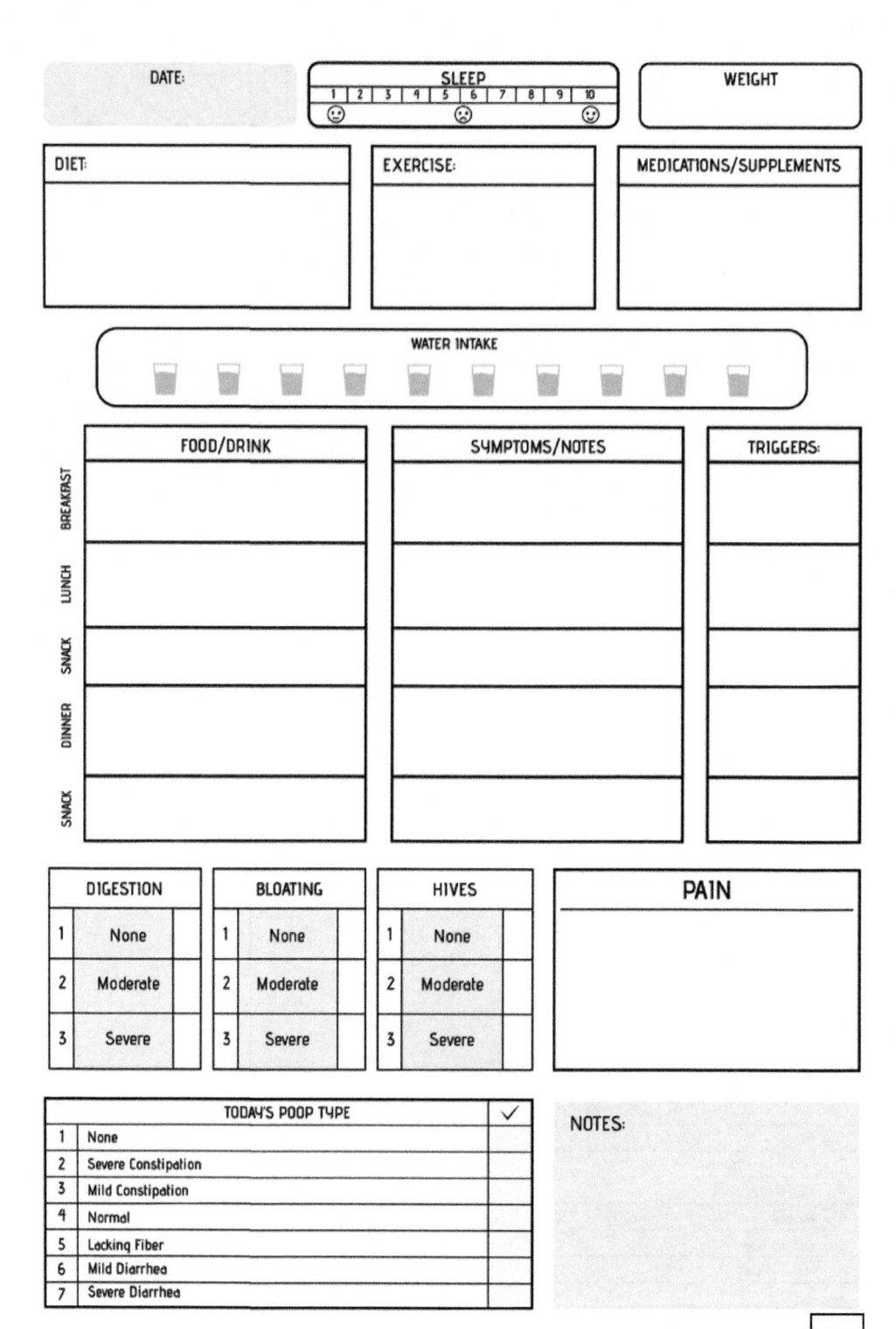

1	2	3	4	5	6	7	8	9	10

DIET:

EXERCISE:

MEDICATIONS/SUPPLEMENTS

WATER INTAKE

FOOD/DRINK	SYMPTOMS/NOTES	TRIGGERS:
BREAKFAST		
LUNCH		
SNACK		
DINNER		
SNACK		

DIGESTION
1	None
2	Moderate
3	Severe

BLOATING
1	None
2	Moderate
3	Severe

HIVES
1	None
2	Moderate
3	Severe

PAIN

TODAY'S POOP TYPE ✓
1	None
2	Severe Constipation
3	Mild Constipation
4	Normal
5	Lacking Fiber
6	Mild Diarrhea
7	Severe Diarrhea

NOTES:

DATE:

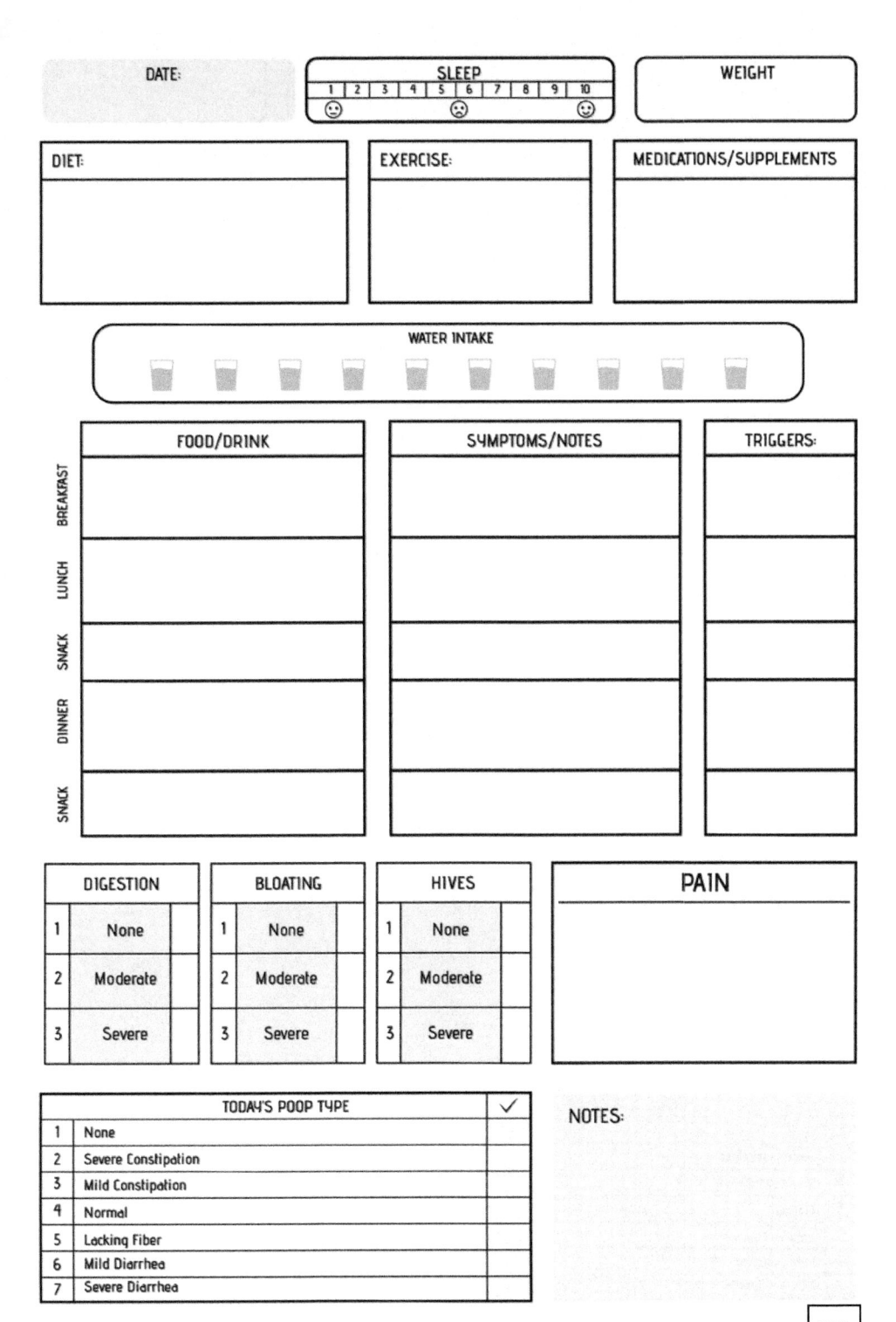

SLEEP
1	2	3	4	5	6	7	8	9	10

☺ ☹ ☺

WEIGHT

DIET:

EXERCISE:

MEDICATIONS/SUPPLEMENTS

WATER INTAKE

	FOOD/DRINK	SYMPTOMS/NOTES	TRIGGERS:
BREAKFAST			
LUNCH			
SNACK			
DINNER			
SNACK			

DIGESTION
1	None
2	Moderate
3	Severe

BLOATING
1	None
2	Moderate
3	Severe

HIVES
1	None
2	Moderate
3	Severe

PAIN

	TODAY'S POOP TYPE	✓
1	None	
2	Severe Constipation	
3	Mild Constipation	
4	Normal	
5	Lacking Fiber	
6	Mild Diarrhea	
7	Severe Diarrhea	

NOTES:

DATE:

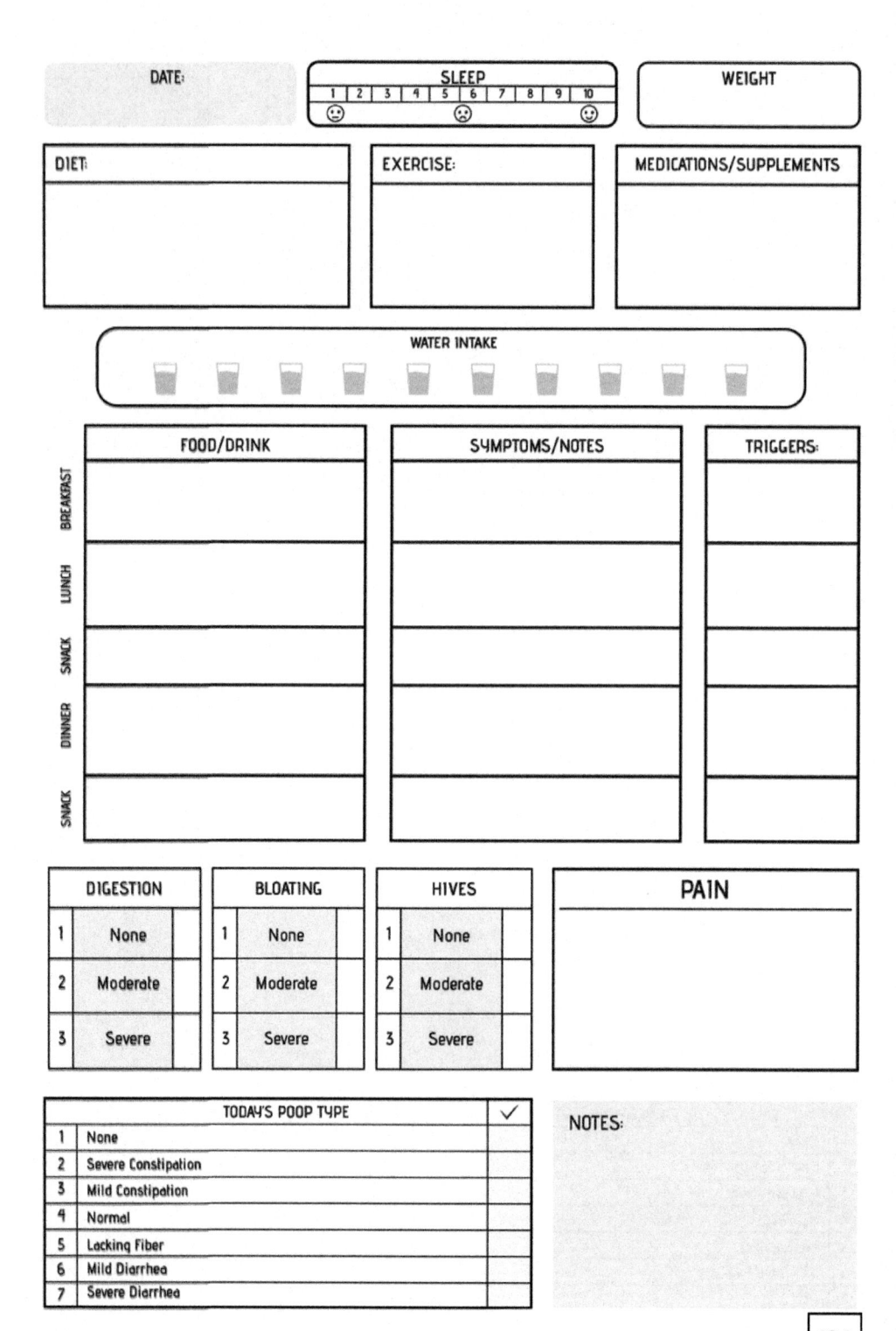

SLEEP
| 1 | 2 | 3 | 4 | 5 | 6 | 7 | 8 | 9 | 10 |

WEIGHT

DIET:

EXERCISE:

MEDICATIONS/SUPPLEMENTS

WATER INTAKE

	FOOD/DRINK	SYMPTOMS/NOTES	TRIGGERS:
BREAKFAST			
LUNCH			
SNACK			
DINNER			
SNACK			

DIGESTION
1	None
2	Moderate
3	Severe

BLOATING
1	None
2	Moderate
3	Severe

HIVES
1	None
2	Moderate
3	Severe

PAIN

TODAY'S POOP TYPE | ✓
1	None
2	Severe Constipation
3	Mild Constipation
4	Normal
5	Lacking Fiber
6	Mild Diarrhea
7	Severe Diarrhea

NOTES:

DATE:

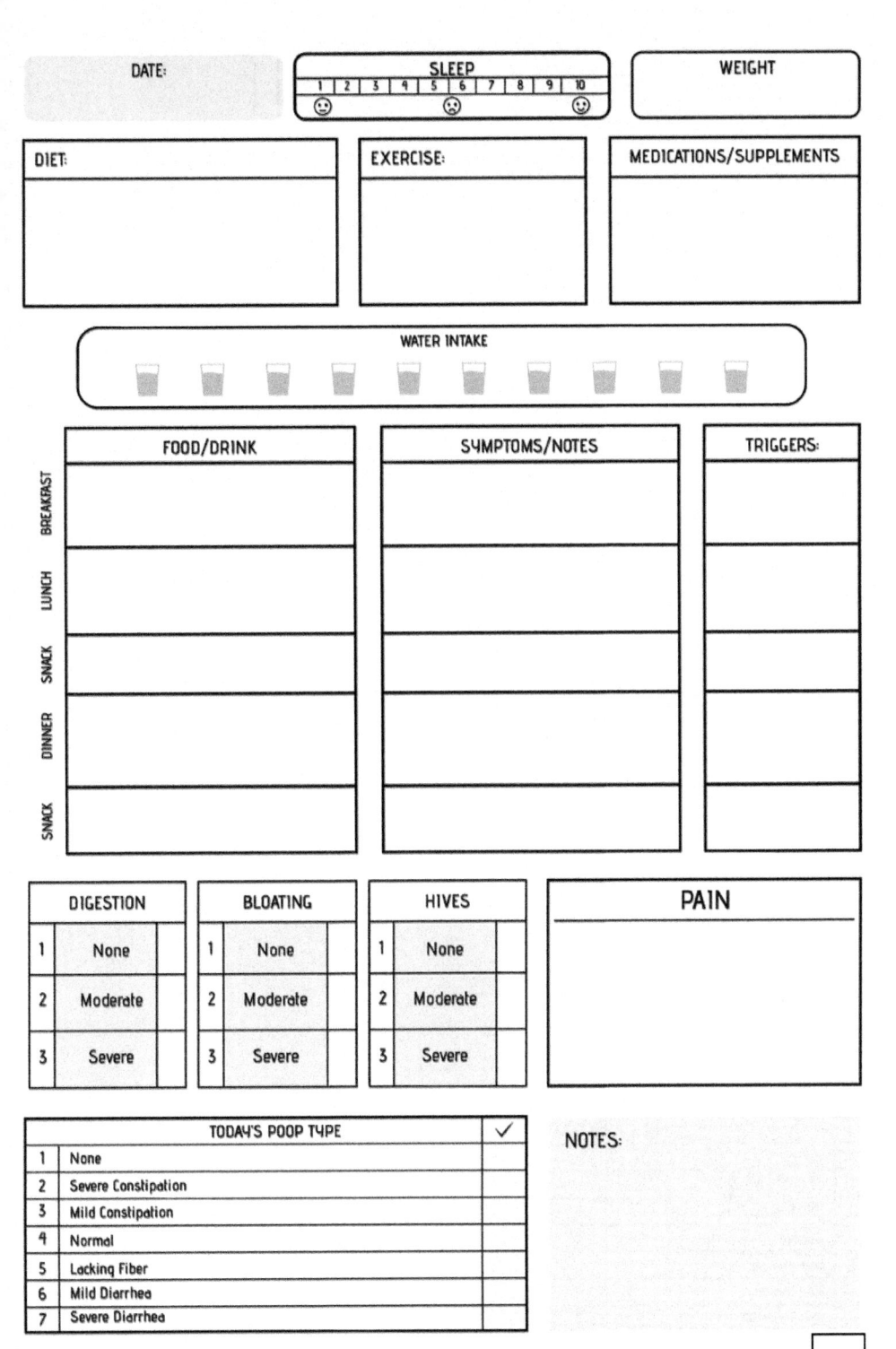

SLEEP
1	2	3	4	5	6	7	8	9	10

WEIGHT

DIET:

EXERCISE:

MEDICATIONS/SUPPLEMENTS

WATER INTAKE

	FOOD/DRINK	SYMPTOMS/NOTES	TRIGGERS:
BREAKFAST			
LUNCH			
SNACK			
DINNER			
SNACK			

DIGESTION
1	None
2	Moderate
3	Severe

BLOATING
1	None
2	Moderate
3	Severe

HIVES
1	None
2	Moderate
3	Severe

PAIN

TODAY'S POOP TYPE ✓
1	None
2	Severe Constipation
3	Mild Constipation
4	Normal
5	Lacking Fiber
6	Mild Diarrhea
7	Severe Diarrhea

NOTES:

DATE:	SLEEP 1 2 3 4 5 6 7 8 9 10	WEIGHT

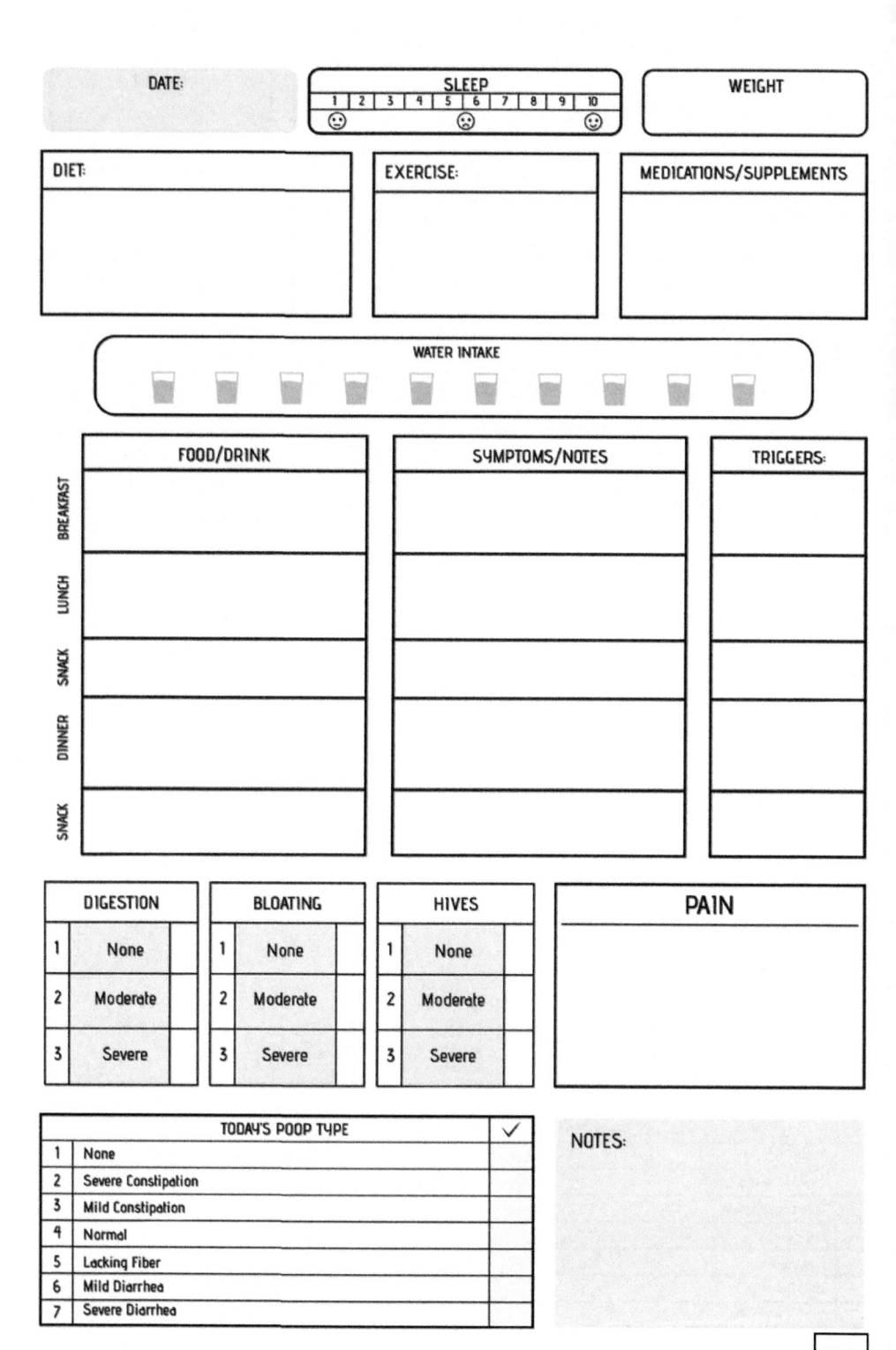

DIET:	EXERCISE:	MEDICATIONS/SUPPLEMENTS

WATER INTAKE

	FOOD/DRINK	SYMPTOMS/NOTES	TRIGGERS:
BREAKFAST			
LUNCH			
SNACK			
DINNER			
SNACK			

DIGESTION		BLOATING		HIVES	
1	None	1	None	1	None
2	Moderate	2	Moderate	2	Moderate
3	Severe	3	Severe	3	Severe

PAIN

	TODAY'S POOP TYPE	✓
1	None	
2	Severe Constipation	
3	Mild Constipation	
4	Normal	
5	Lacking Fiber	
6	Mild Diarrhea	
7	Severe Diarrhea	

NOTES:

DATE:

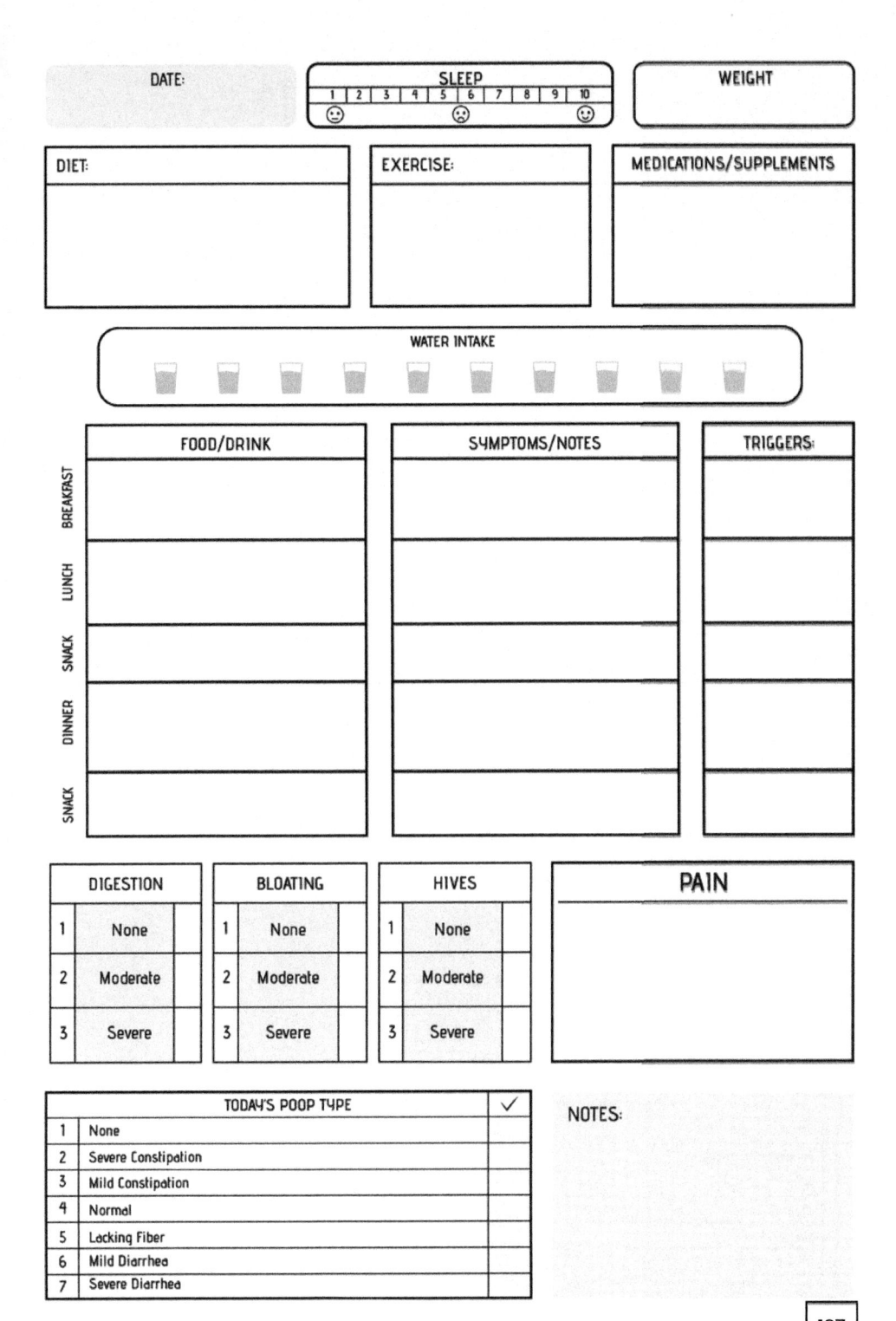

SLEEP | 1 | 2 | 3 | 4 | 5 | 6 | 7 | 8 | 9 | 10

WEIGHT

DIET:

EXERCISE:

MEDICATIONS/SUPPLEMENTS

WATER INTAKE

	FOOD/DRINK	SYMPTOMS/NOTES	TRIGGERS:
BREAKFAST			
LUNCH			
SNACK			
DINNER			
SNACK			

DIGESTION		BLOATING		HIVES	
1	None	1	None	1	None
2	Moderate	2	Moderate	2	Moderate
3	Severe	3	Severe	3	Severe

PAIN

	TODAY'S POOP TYPE	✓
1	None	
2	Severe Constipation	
3	Mild Constipation	
4	Normal	
5	Lacking Fiber	
6	Mild Diarrhea	
7	Severe Diarrhea	

NOTES:

DATE:

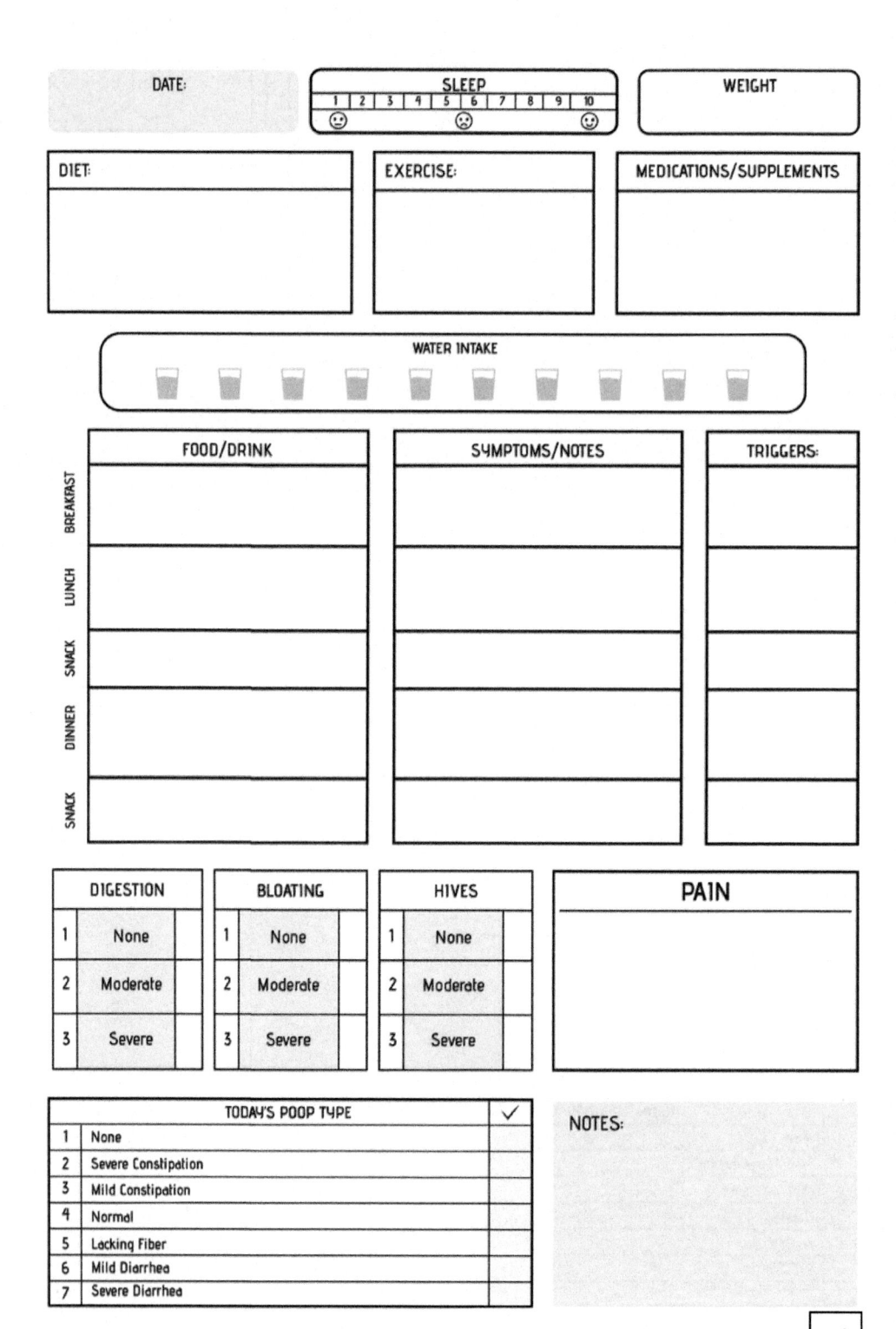

SLEEP
1	2	3	4	5	6	7	8	9	10

WEIGHT

DIET:

EXERCISE:

MEDICATIONS/SUPPLEMENTS

WATER INTAKE

	FOOD/DRINK	SYMPTOMS/NOTES	TRIGGERS:
BREAKFAST			
LUNCH			
SNACK			
DINNER			
SNACK			

DIGESTION
1	None
2	Moderate
3	Severe

BLOATING
1	None
2	Moderate
3	Severe

HIVES
1	None
2	Moderate
3	Severe

PAIN

TODAY'S POOP TYPE ✓
1	None
2	Severe Constipation
3	Mild Constipation
4	Normal
5	Lacking Fiber
6	Mild Diarrhea
7	Severe Diarrhea

NOTES:

DATE:

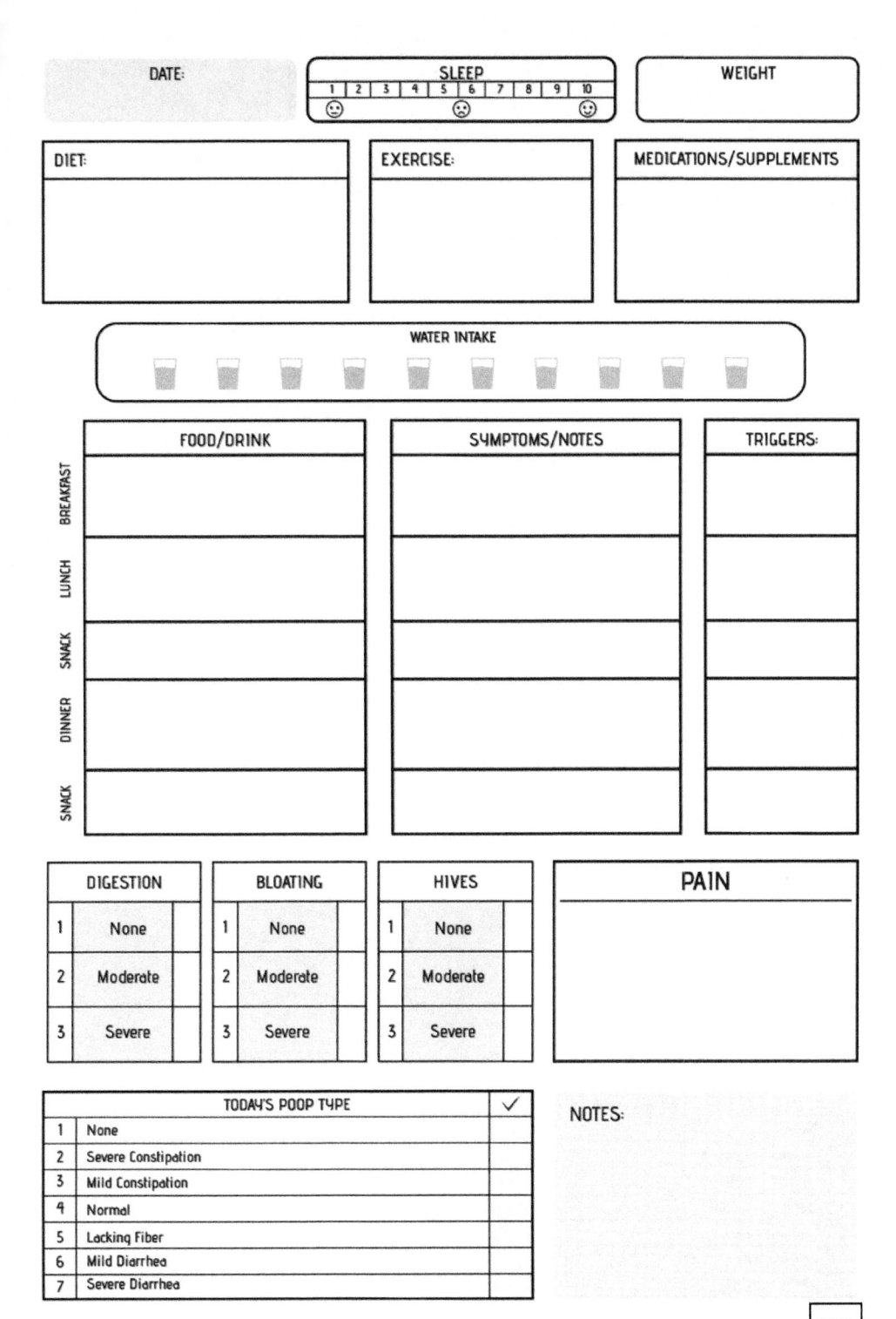

SLEEP 1 2 3 4 5 6 7 8 9 10

WEIGHT

DIET:

EXERCISE:

MEDICATIONS/SUPPLEMENTS

WATER INTAKE

	FOOD/DRINK	SYMPTOMS/NOTES	TRIGGERS:
BREAKFAST			
LUNCH			
SNACK			
DINNER			
SNACK			

DIGESTION		BLOATING		HIVES	
1	None	1	None	1	None
2	Moderate	2	Moderate	2	Moderate
3	Severe	3	Severe	3	Severe

PAIN

	TODAY'S POOP TYPE	✓
1	None	
2	Severe Constipation	
3	Mild Constipation	
4	Normal	
5	Lacking Fiber	
6	Mild Diarrhea	
7	Severe Diarrhea	

NOTES:

DATE:

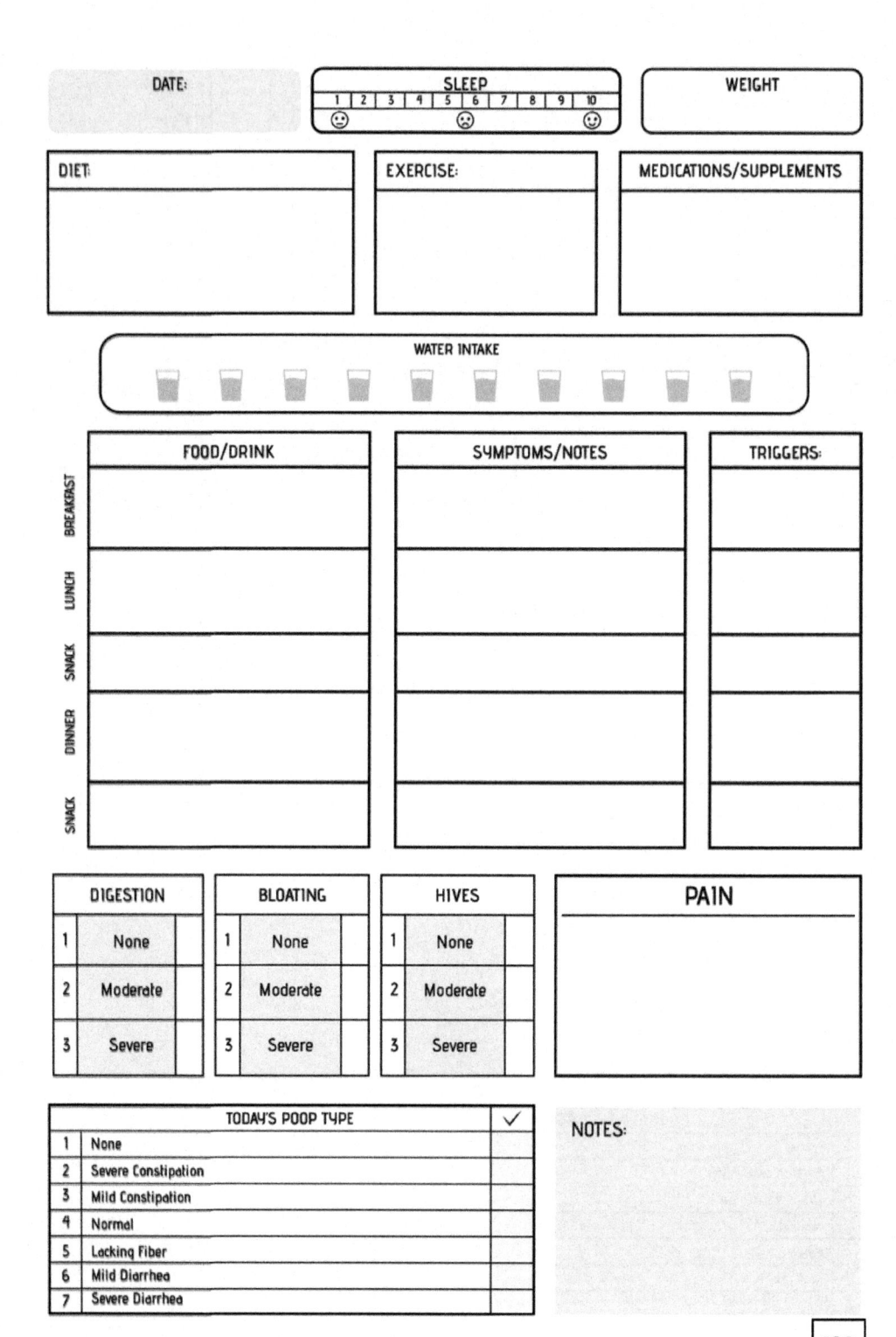

SLEEP
1	2	3	4	5	6	7	8	9	10

WEIGHT

DIET:

EXERCISE:

MEDICATIONS/SUPPLEMENTS

WATER INTAKE

	FOOD/DRINK	SYMPTOMS/NOTES	TRIGGERS:
BREAKFAST			
LUNCH			
SNACK			
DINNER			
SNACK			

DIGESTION
1	None
2	Moderate
3	Severe

BLOATING
1	None
2	Moderate
3	Severe

HIVES
1	None
2	Moderate
3	Severe

PAIN

TODAY'S POOP TYPE ✓
1	None
2	Severe Constipation
3	Mild Constipation
4	Normal
5	Lacking Fiber
6	Mild Diarrhea
7	Severe Diarrhea

NOTES:

DATE:

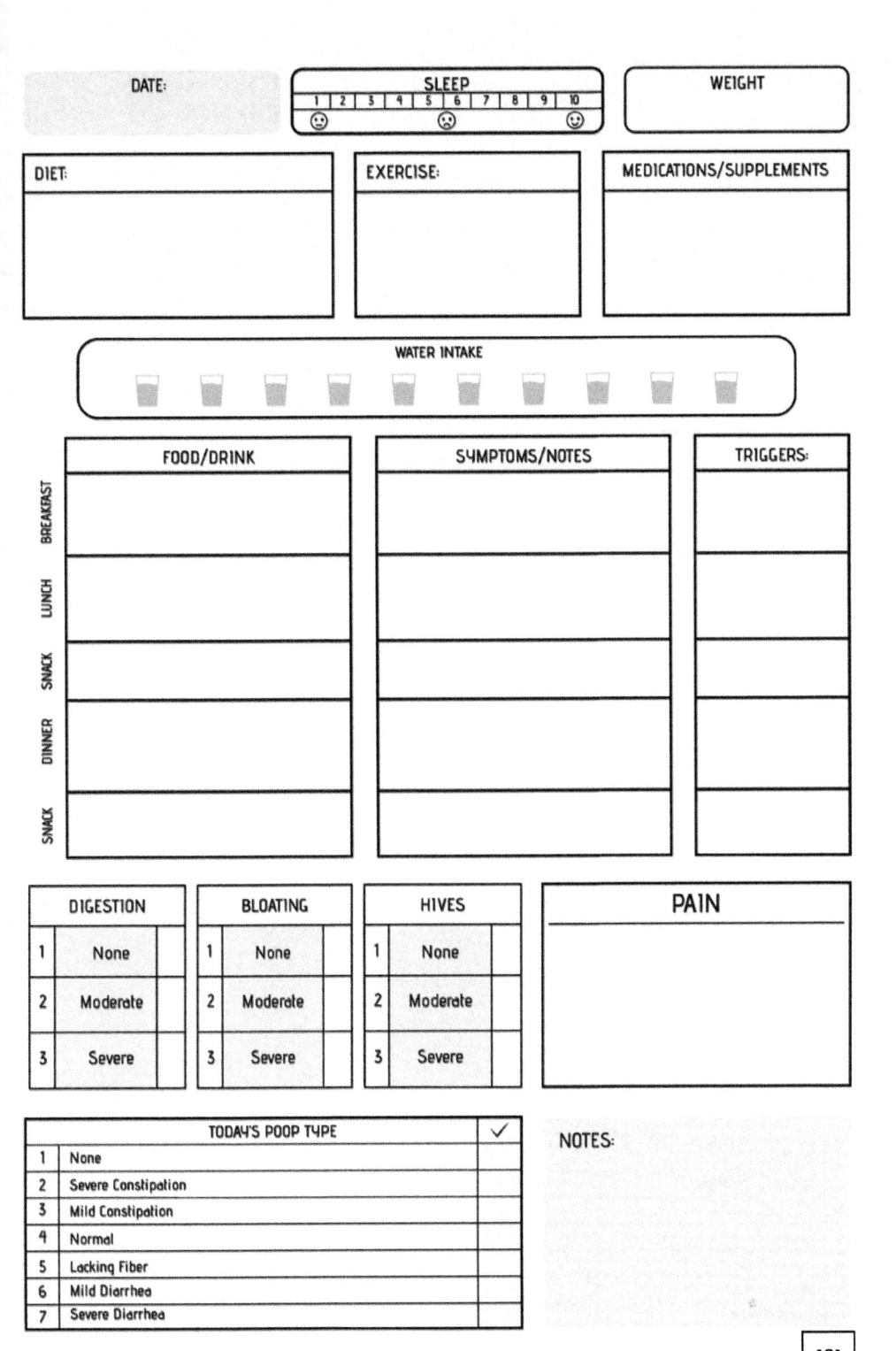

SLEEP 1 2 3 4 5 6 7 8 9 10

WEIGHT

DIET:

EXERCISE:

MEDICATIONS/SUPPLEMENTS

WATER INTAKE

	FOOD/DRINK	SYMPTOMS/NOTES	TRIGGERS:
BREAKFAST			
LUNCH			
SNACK			
DINNER			
SNACK			

	DIGESTION
1	None
2	Moderate
3	Severe

	BLOATING
1	None
2	Moderate
3	Severe

	HIVES
1	None
2	Moderate
3	Severe

PAIN

	TODAY'S POOP TYPE	✓
1	None	
2	Severe Constipation	
3	Mild Constipation	
4	Normal	
5	Lacking Fiber	
6	Mild Diarrhea	
7	Severe Diarrhea	

NOTES:

DATE:

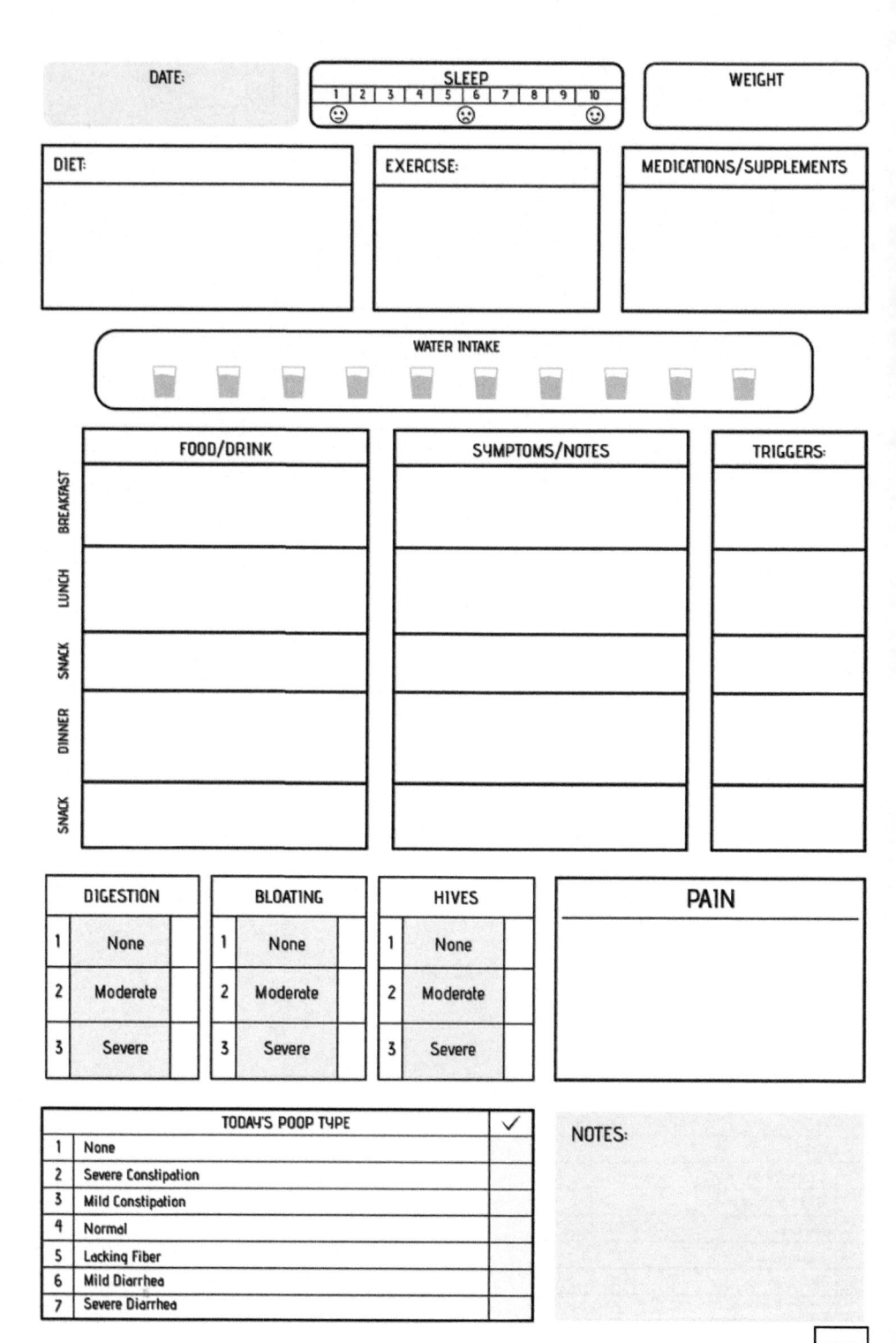

SLEEP
1	2	3	4	5	6	7	8	9	10

WEIGHT

DIET:

EXERCISE:

MEDICATIONS/SUPPLEMENTS

WATER INTAKE

	FOOD/DRINK	SYMPTOMS/NOTES	TRIGGERS:
BREAKFAST			
LUNCH			
SNACK			
DINNER			
SNACK			

DIGESTION			BLOATING			HIVES	
1	None		1	None		1	None
2	Moderate		2	Moderate		2	Moderate
3	Severe		3	Severe		3	Severe

PAIN

	TODAY'S POOP TYPE	✓
1	None	
2	Severe Constipation	
3	Mild Constipation	
4	Normal	
5	Lacking Fiber	
6	Mild Diarrhea	
7	Severe Diarrhea	

NOTES:

DATE:

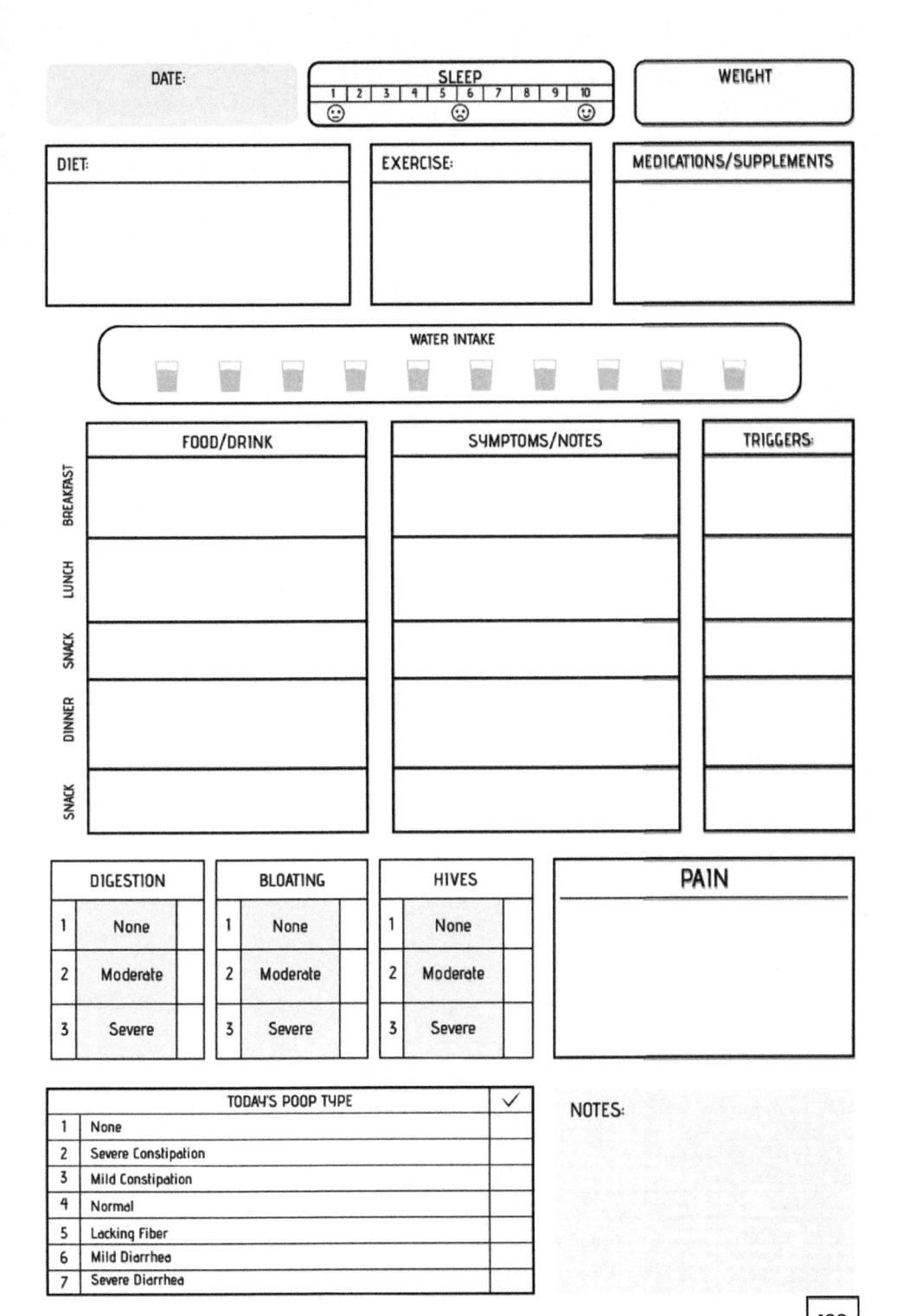

SLEEP
| 1 | 2 | 3 | 4 | 5 | 6 | 7 | 8 | 9 | 10 |

WEIGHT

DIET:

EXERCISE:

MEDICATIONS/SUPPLEMENTS

WATER INTAKE

FOOD/DRINK	SYMPTOMS/NOTES	TRIGGERS:
BREAKFAST		
LUNCH		
SNACK		
DINNER		
SNACK		

DIGESTION
1	None
2	Moderate
3	Severe

BLOATING
1	None
2	Moderate
3	Severe

HIVES
1	None
2	Moderate
3	Severe

PAIN

	TODAY'S POOP TYPE	✓
1	None	
2	Severe Constipation	
3	Mild Constipation	
4	Normal	
5	Lacking Fiber	
6	Mild Diarrhea	
7	Severe Diarrhea	

NOTES:

DATE:

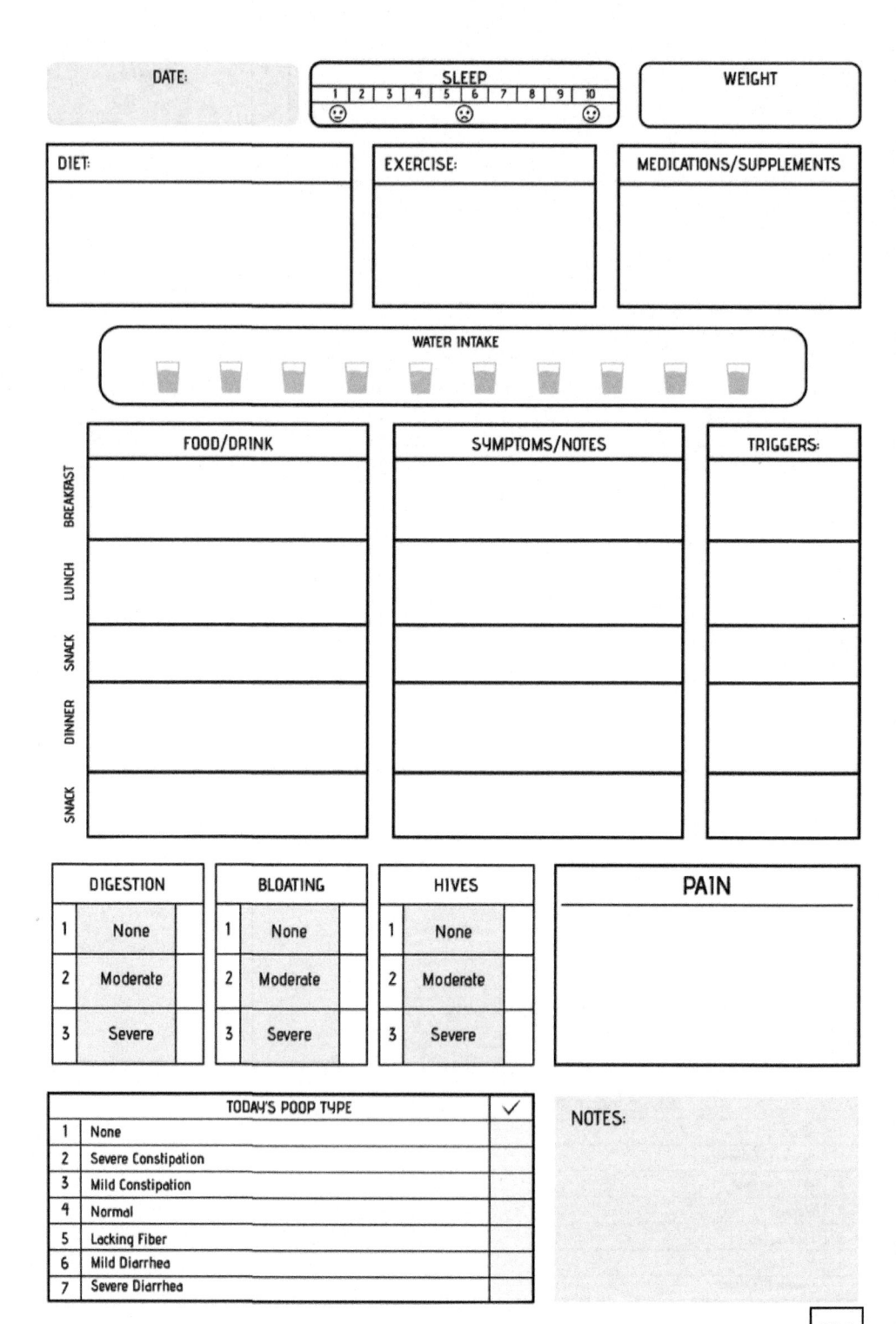

SLEEP
1	2	3	4	5	6	7	8	9	10

WEIGHT

DIET:

EXERCISE:

MEDICATIONS/SUPPLEMENTS

WATER INTAKE

	FOOD/DRINK	SYMPTOMS/NOTES	TRIGGERS:
BREAKFAST			
LUNCH			
SNACK			
DINNER			
SNACK			

DIGESTION
1	None
2	Moderate
3	Severe

BLOATING
1	None
2	Moderate
3	Severe

HIVES
1	None
2	Moderate
3	Severe

PAIN

TODAY'S POOP TYPE ✓
1	None
2	Severe Constipation
3	Mild Constipation
4	Normal
5	Lacking Fiber
6	Mild Diarrhea
7	Severe Diarrhea

NOTES:

134

| DATE: | SLEEP 1 2 3 4 5 6 7 8 9 10 | WEIGHT |

| DIET: | EXERCISE: | MEDICATIONS/SUPPLEMENTS |

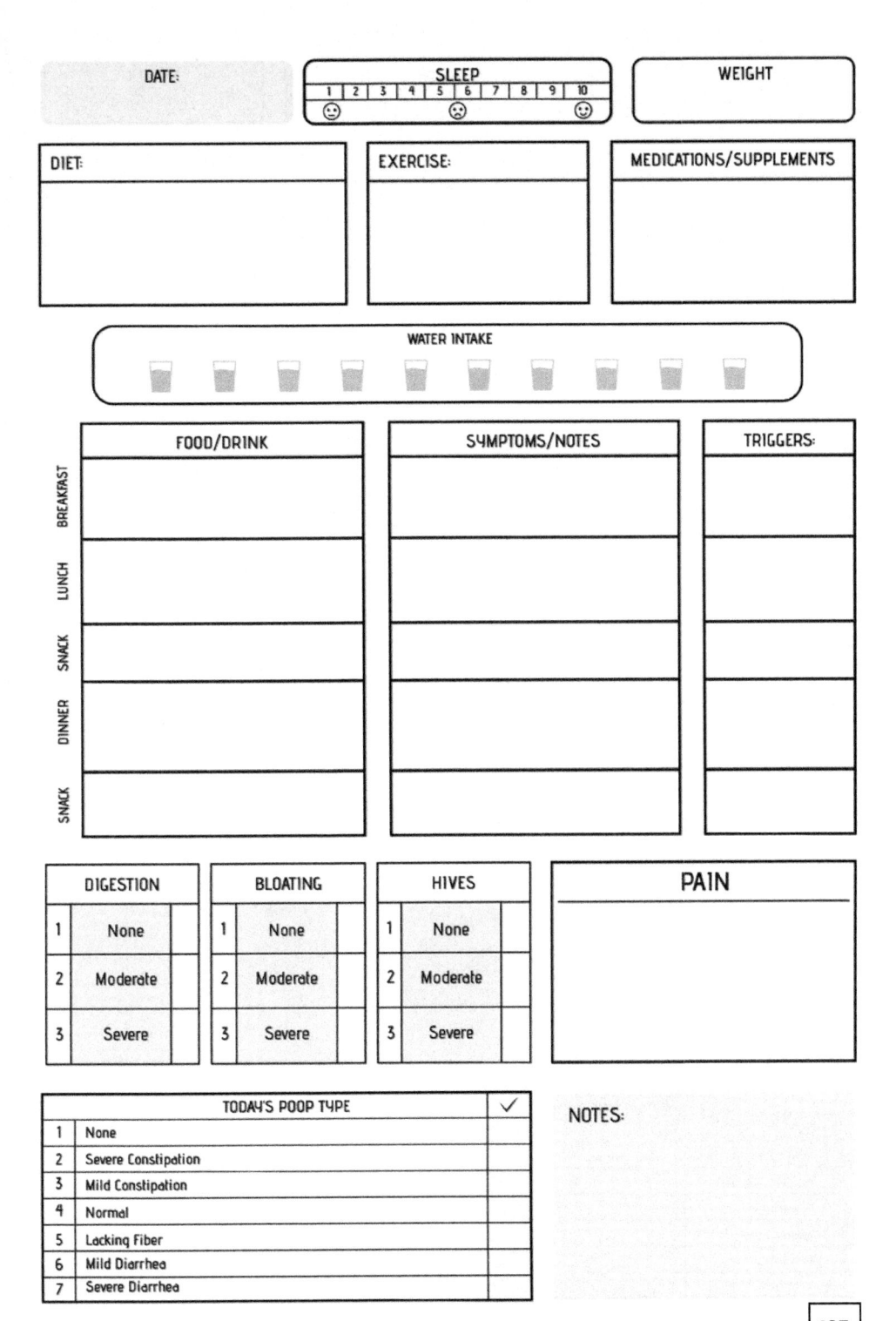

WATER INTAKE

	FOOD/DRINK	SYMPTOMS/NOTES	TRIGGERS:
BREAKFAST			
LUNCH			
SNACK			
DINNER			
SNACK			

DIGESTION		BLOATING		HIVES	
1	None	1	None	1	None
2	Moderate	2	Moderate	2	Moderate
3	Severe	3	Severe	3	Severe

PAIN

#	TODAY'S POOP TYPE	✓
1	None	
2	Severe Constipation	
3	Mild Constipation	
4	Normal	
5	Lacking Fiber	
6	Mild Diarrhea	
7	Severe Diarrhea	

NOTES:

DATE:

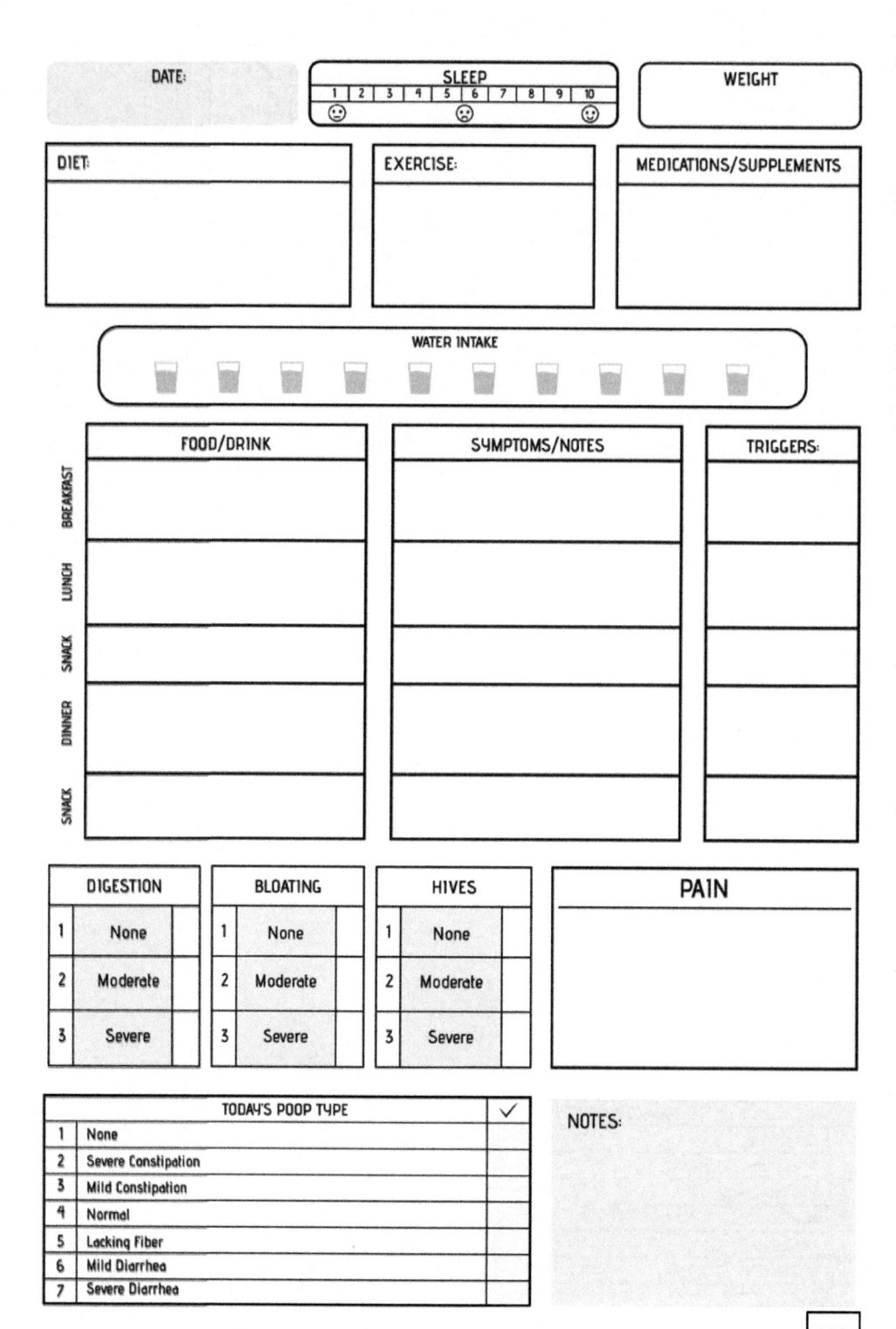

SLEEP
1	2	3	4	5	6	7	8	9	10

WEIGHT

DIET:

EXERCISE:

MEDICATIONS/SUPPLEMENTS

WATER INTAKE

	FOOD/DRINK	SYMPTOMS/NOTES	TRIGGERS:
BREAKFAST			
LUNCH			
SNACK			
DINNER			
SNACK			

DIGESTION
1	None
2	Moderate
3	Severe

BLOATING
1	None
2	Moderate
3	Severe

HIVES
1	None
2	Moderate
3	Severe

PAIN

TODAY'S POOP TYPE | ✓
1	None	
2	Severe Constipation	
3	Mild Constipation	
4	Normal	
5	Lacking Fiber	
6	Mild Diarrhea	
7	Severe Diarrhea	

NOTES:

DATE:

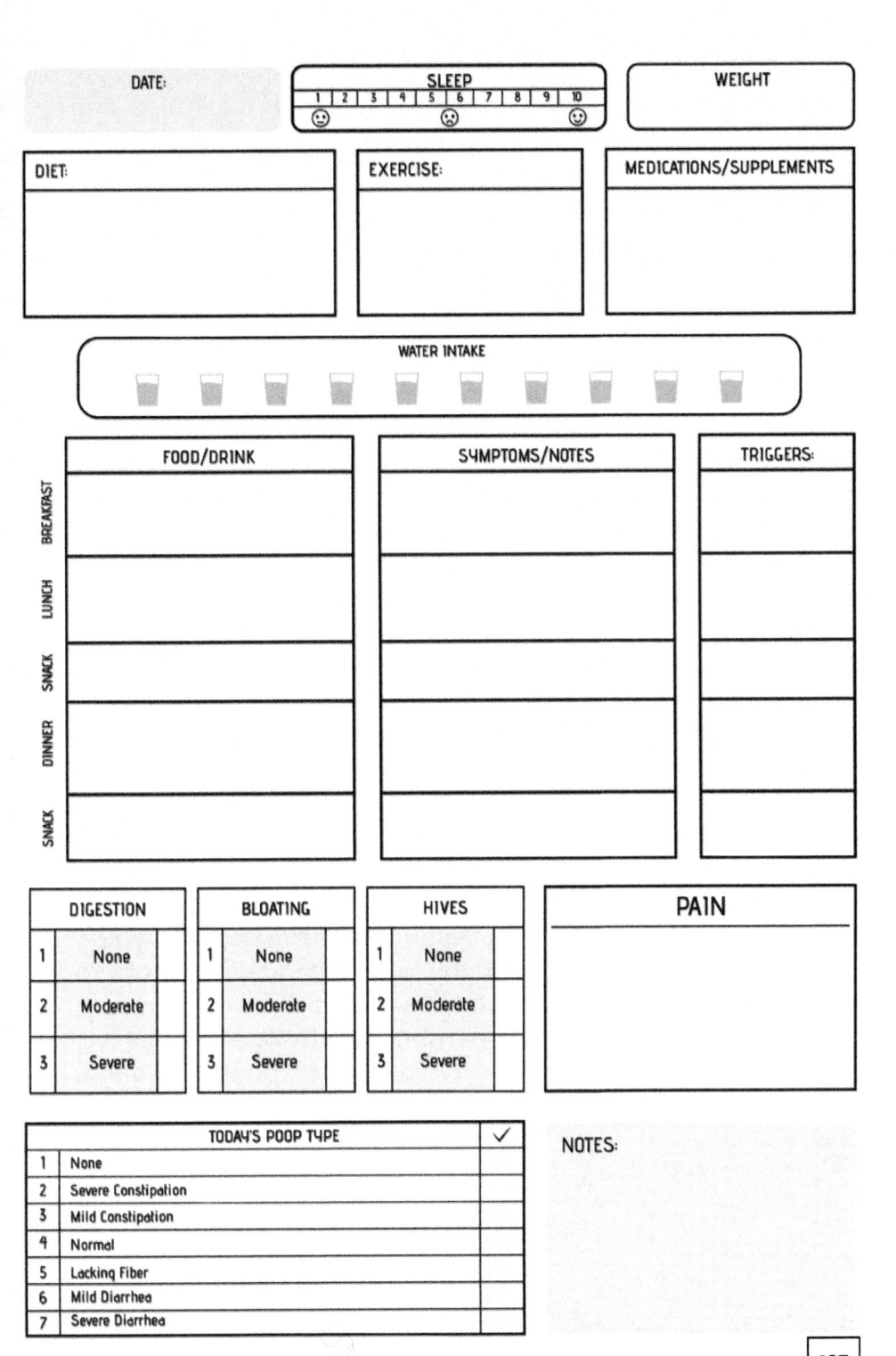

SLEEP | 1 | 2 | 3 | 4 | 5 | 6 | 7 | 8 | 9 | 10

WEIGHT

DIET:

EXERCISE:

MEDICATIONS/SUPPLEMENTS

WATER INTAKE

	FOOD/DRINK	SYMPTOMS/NOTES	TRIGGERS:
BREAKFAST			
LUNCH			
SNACK			
DINNER			
SNACK			

DIGESTION		BLOATING		HIVES	
1	None	1	None	1	None
2	Moderate	2	Moderate	2	Moderate
3	Severe	3	Severe	3	Severe

PAIN

	TODAY'S POOP TYPE	✓
1	None	
2	Severe Constipation	
3	Mild Constipation	
4	Normal	
5	Lacking Fiber	
6	Mild Diarrhea	
7	Severe Diarrhea	

NOTES:

How to Interpret Your Progress:

- Score Improvements: Look for gradual increases in scores each week, suggesting positive impacts from the low FODMAP diet on aspects like digestive comfort or energy levels.
- Understanding Your Body's Responses: Consistent patterns in your scores can reveal which areas benefit most from the diet and which might need different strategies or more attention.
- Identifying Patterns: Connecting your diet to overall well-being is key. Notice how dietary changes might influence different health aspects, like mood or sleep.
- Considering Limitations: Keep in mind that these scores are subjective and can be influenced by external factors like stress, lifestyle changes, or physical activity.
- Reflecting on Your Journey: At the end of the 28 days, review your overall progress. Look beyond the scores to consider emotional and physical feelings throughout the plan. Use these insights to learn what dietary habits worked best for you and how you might want to continue adapting your diet.

By consistently tracking and reflecting on these aspects, you'll gain valuable insights into how the low FODMAP diet affects your body, helping you make more informed decisions about your long-term dietary choices. Remember, this table serves as a guide to help you understand your body's unique responses to dietary changes.

SECTION 4: WHAT NEXT

Remember the key quote....

The low FODMAP diet is a temporary eating plan that's very restrictive

As you reach the end of your structured 28-day low FODMAP journey, you've undoubtedly gained valuable insights into how different foods influence your gut health. But what comes next is equally crucial.

The careful reintroduction of foods. This phase is key to understanding your unique dietary triggers and forging a long-term eating plan that keeps your symptoms at bay.

THE 6 STEPS

1. Gradual Reintroduction:

- **Why Start Slowly:** Introducing high FODMAP foods one at a time is essential for identifying which specific foods trigger your symptoms. If you reintroduce multiple foods simultaneously, it becomes difficult to pinpoint which food is responsible for any potential flare-up. The goal is to achieve a clear understanding of your food tolerances.
- **How to Begin:** Start with one high FODMAP food you used to enjoy or one that offers nutritional benefits you've been missing. Introduce this food in a small amount, and monitor how your body reacts over the next 24-48 hours.
- **Controlled Portions:**
  - **Why Controlled Portions:** The quantity of a high FODMAP food can significantly impact your body's response. A small amount might not trigger symptoms, while a larger serving could. Controlled portions help determine your tolerance level to different FODMAPs.
  - **How to Implement:** Begin with a small serving of the reintroduced food - for example, a half slice of regular bread or a few pieces of an apple. If you don't experience any adverse symptoms, you can gradually increase the portion size over subsequent days. This step-by-step approach allows your digestive system to adjust without being overwhelmed.

2. Monitor Your Responses:

Monitoring your responses during the reintroduction phase of the FODMAP diet can be likened to structuring a revision strategy for a test. Just as you would organize and assess your study material to understand which areas you're strong in and which need more attention, you should similarly structure your approach to reintroducing foods. Here's how you can apply this analogy:

Structured Approach
- Creating a Plan: Just as you would create a study schedule before a test, plan which high FODMAP foods to reintroduce and when. Start with foods you're most interested in or that offer nutritional benefits you've been missing.
- One at a Time: Like focusing on one subject at a time to avoid confusion and overlap, reintroduce one food at a time. This methodical approach helps in clearly identifying how each specific food affects your symptoms.

Careful Observation
- Tracking Responses: As you would note down key points or areas of difficulty while studying, keep a detailed record of how your body reacts to each reintroduced food. Note down any changes in symptoms, no matter how small.
- Adjusting as Needed: Just as you might adjust your study plan based on areas where you feel less confident, adjust your diet based on your body's reactions. If a food consistently triggers symptoms, consider limiting it or removing it from your diet.

Evaluating Progress
- Review Regularly: Like periodically reviewing your study notes to gauge your understanding, regularly assess your food diary. Look for patterns or trends – which foods are well-tolerated, and which are not.
- Making Informed Decisions: In the same way that a practice test helps you decide what to focus on in your final revision, use the insights from your food diary to make informed decisions about your long-term diet.

3. Seek Variety:

Nutritional Balance:
- Comprehensive Nutrition: Each food group offers unique nutrients vital for overall health. By gradually reintroducing different food groups, you ensure your body receives a full spectrum of nutrients. This includes essential vitamins, minerals, antioxidants, and fibers that are key to maintaining good health.
- Preventing Nutritional Deficiencies: Sticking solely to low FODMAP foods can sometimes limit your intake of certain nutrients. By reintroducing various foods, you minimize the risk of deficiencies and promote a more balanced diet.

Expanding Food Choices:
- Discovering Tolerances: The reintroduction phase helps identify which high FODMAP foods you can tolerate, allowing you to reintroduce these into your diet. This discovery can significantly broaden your food choices.
- Culinary Exploration: With each successfully reintroduced food, you open up new possibilities for recipes and meals. This makes your diet more interesting and enjoyable, which is important for long-term adherence to healthy eating habits.
- **Emotional and Social Benefits:** Eating a wider variety of foods also has emotional and social benefits. Being able to participate more fully in social meals and enjoy a broader range of culinary experiences can significantly improve your quality of life.

In this phase, it's crucial to continue monitoring your body's reactions and adjust your diet accordingly. By doing so, you create a personalized eating plan that balances the management of your symptoms with a rich, varied, and enjoyable diet. This approach not only addresses your immediate dietary needs but also sets the foundation for a sustainable and healthful eating pattern in the long term.

4. Listen to Your Body:
- **Adjusting to Tolerance:** Recognize that your body's response to different foods is unique. What may be tolerable for others might not suit you. Observe how your body reacts to each reintroduced food and adjust your diet accordingly. This process is not about adhering strictly to a set list but about understanding and respecting your body's signals.
- **Patience is Key:** Just as it takes time to learn a new skill, it takes time for your body to adjust to dietary changes. Be patient with yourself as you navigate this new dietary landscape. Some foods may need to be reintroduced multiple times to accurately gauge your tolerance levels.

5. Consult Healthcare Professionals:
- **Seek Expert Guidance:** Navigating the complexities of food reintroduction can be challenging. If you find yourself unsure or overwhelmed, don't hesitate to seek advice from a dietitian or healthcare provider. They can provide clarity and direction, ensuring you're on the right track.
- **Tailored Advice for Individual Needs:** Healthcare professionals can offer personalized guidance based on your specific health condition, dietary needs, and progress. Their expert insights can be invaluable in fine-tuning your diet for optimal results.

6. Long-term Management:
- **Adopting a Flexible Approach:** The ultimate goal is to develop a diet that is both enjoyable and conducive to your health. This might mean having a diet that includes a balance of low and high FODMAP foods, depending on your individual tolerance levels.
- **Periodic Review and Adjustment:** Just as life changes, so too can your body's needs and reactions. Regularly reviewing and adjusting your diet is crucial. This ongoing process ensures that your diet continues to align with your health objectives and lifestyle changes.

FODMAP RESOURCE GUIDE

Welcome to the bonus section tailored for your FODMAP-friendly journey! This compilation of resources is designed to enhance your knowledge and support, catering to diverse interests - from avid readers to digital content enthusiasts.

Enlightening Reads:
- "The Complete Low-FODMAP Diet" by Sue Shepherd and Peter Gibson: This book serves as a comprehensive guide, providing a deep dive into managing IBS and other digestive conditions through a low-FODMAP diet. It's packed with scientific insights and practical tips.
- "The Low-FODMAP Diet Step by Step" by Kate Scarlata and Dede Wilson: This is a practical and visually appealing guide, offering a step-by-step approach to adopting a low FODMAP diet, including recipes and dietary tips.
- "IBS-Free at Last!" by Patsy Catsos: This book offers a personal and insightful look into managing IBS with a FODMAP-focused approach. Catsos combines personal experiences with professional expertise, making it a relatable and informative read.
- "The FODMAP Navigator" by Martin Storr: A great resource for those seeking a quick reference guide to FODMAPs, this book offers lists of foods categorized by their FODMAP content, helping you navigate your diet more easily.

Podcasts for Your Listening Pleasure:
- "The IBS Freedom Podcast" hosted by Nikki DuBose and Amy Hollenkamp: This podcast covers a range of topics around IBS and the low FODMAP diet, blending expert insights with personal experiences.
- "FODMAP Stories" by Larah Brook: A podcast that shares personal stories of those managing a low FODMAP diet, offering encouragement and practical advice.

Screen Time with FODMAP:
- "Monash FODMAP" YouTube Channel: From the creators of the Monash University FODMAP Diet App, this channel provides scientifically backed information, cooking tips, and educational content on FODMAPs.

- Documentary Series: Look for documentaries focused on gut health, IBS, and nutritional wellness. They often cover aspects of the low FODMAP diet as part of broader discussions on digestive health.

YouTube Channels: Visual Learning and Support:
- "FODMAP Formula" YouTube Channel: This channel offers practical advice on following a low FODMAP diet, including recipe tutorials and shopping tips.
- "Fun Without FODMAPs" YouTube Channel: Focuses on creating delicious and varied low FODMAP recipes, perfect for those looking to expand their culinary repertoire while managing dietary restrictions.

Each of these resources provides valuable insights and varied perspectives on managing a low FODMAP diet. Whether you're curled up with an informative book, listening to inspiring stories on a podcast, or engaging with educational videos, these resources will enrich your journey and support you in navigating the FODMAP landscape effectively. Enjoy your exploration and discovery on this path to better digestive health!

THANK YOU NOTE

I would like to extend a heartfelt thank you for embarking on this journey through the pages of this guide. Your commitment to understanding and managing your dietary needs, especially in navigating the low FODMAP landscape, is commendable. This journey, no doubt, requires patience, perseverance, and a willingness to learn and adapt. Your dedication to improving your health and well-being is truly inspiring. Remember, every step you've taken is a stride towards better health and a more comfortable life. May the knowledge you've gained here continue to guide and support you on your

BNW
PUBLISH

Join us on your favourite platform, Scan the QR code on your phone or tablet

THANK YOU

please review on amazon

★★★★★

Printed in Great Britain
by Amazon